Arthritis Begone!

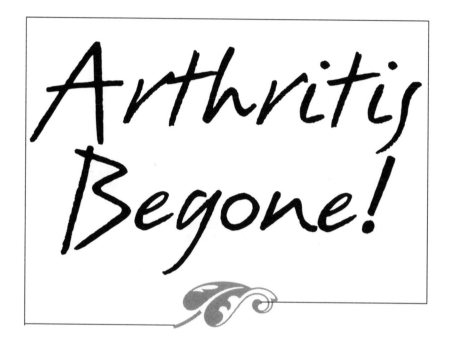

Arthritis Begone!

A Doctor's ℞ for Easy, Safe
Inexpensive—and Effective—Treatments
for Your Arthritis Pain

JOHN B. IRWIN, M.D.

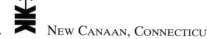

KEATS PUBLISHING, INC.   NEW CANAAN, CONNECTICUT

Arthritis Begone! is intended solely as information and education, and not as medical advice. Please consult a medical or health professional if you have questions about your health.

ARTHRITIS BEGONE!
Copyright © 1997 by John B. Irwin
All Rights Reserved

Library of Congress Cataloging-in-Publication Data

Irwin, John B.
    Arthritis begone! : a doctor's ℞ for easy, safe, inexpensive—
and effective—treatments for your arthritis pain / John B. Irwin.
        p.   cm.
    Includes bibliographical references and index.
    ISBN 0-87983-804-3
    1. Arthritis—Popular works.   2. Arthritis—Treatment.   I. Title.
RC933.I78   1997
616.7'22—dc21   97-25611
                                                                       CIP

Printed in the United States of America

Keats Publishing, Inc.
27 Pine Street (Box 876)
New Canaan, Connecticut 06840-0876

Keats Publishing website address: www.keats.com

Contents

Arthritis Begone!

1
Getting Better

AN INTRODUCTION TO LIVING WITH ARTHRITIS

ARE YOU one of the 38,000,000 or more Americans who are suffering from some form of arthritis? Are you among the multitude of patients who have spent a fortune on arthritis treatments without experiencing any significant relief? Would you be interested in alternative measures that are highly effective at much less cost and with essentially no danger? If your answer is "Yes!" to any of these questions, read on. This book will teach you in simple laymen's terms what arthritis is all about and how you can manage your own arthritis condition, using my innovative and well-tested system. No other book or program exists that can give you the same unified information, or the same realistic hopes for marked arthritis relief.

Let me say at the outset that I am not a specialist in rheumatology, the area of medicine devoted to arthritis and the more than 100 inflammatory diseases of joints and soft tissues that this term encompasses. I am, rather, a board-certified obstetrician-gynecologist who has practiced as a physician-surgeon for over 40 years. Despite being technically an outsider when it comes to arthritis, I became extremely interested in rheumatic diseases beginning about thirty years ago as the direct result of the gradual worsening of my own arthritis condition. My interest as a physician was further stimulated when I began to notice that some of my gynecological patients, coincident with undergoing hormone replacement therapy during menopause, experienced a significant improvement in arthritis symptoms. Stiffness, pain and swelling were all reduced; sometimes, they disappeared altogether! This suggested to me that there might be some cause-and-effect clues to arthritis that were currently being overlooked and might be worth further exploration. I began to delve more extensively in medical libraries to see if anyone else was following the same clues. What I found surprised me. No one had paid attention to what were, in my mind, certain obvious causes and effects in arthritis. Indeed, when I compared my own experiences with what was written, I found a lot of "expert knowledge" to be, frankly, wrong or incomplete.

Over time, I have developed new and admittedly unorthodox hypotheses about the nature and causes of the diseases known broadly as arthritis. From these hypotheses have evolved a number of successful treatment approaches that are simple as they are safe. In many cases, you can adopt them without a physician's prescription because they involve such self-determined changes as altering the foods you eat and the kinds of exercises you follow. Perhaps their ultra-simplicity is one factor in physicians' resistance to trying them on patients in their own practices: "How could anything so simple be the answer to a disease so complex?" they seemed to be saying. But then, professional resistance to virtually all forms of alternative medicine today is massive! Recognizing these obstacles, but convinced that I can help many to help themselves, I have decided to go directly to you, the public, with my treatment, and let you judge for yourself through your own knowledge and experience.

Many of you will be familiar with Dr. Jason Theodosakis's very popular book *The Arthritis Cure*, and wonder if this work isn't more of the same. It is not. Like me, Dr. Theodosakis was severely afflicted with arthritis and threw himself into a highly motivated search for an alternative to the standard treatment. And, like me, he discovered something that restored him to normal health and activity. For him it was a course of treatment with several components, based on the use of the supplements glucosamine sulfate and chondroitin sulfate; and he recounts many successes with patients. Comparing the results he obtained with my own experience with more than 1000 patients leaves me persuaded that my system is more logical, complete and effective, though I cannot claim it is a cure, since, even when 100 percent relief of symptoms is obtained, the treatment responsible for that success has to be maintained. As it happens, I do use glucosamine in my therapy, as a useful but minor adjunct.

Of course, no treatment is absolutely effective for everyone; and, conversely, few are not effective for someone. Dr. Theodosakis and I were each fortunate in discovering what worked for us, and naturally wished to share the benefits of our discoveries with the public. Many have benefited from what Dr. Theodosakis recommends; the same is true of my treatment, which seems to me to be rather more successful, both in the number of people helped and the extent of relief. And I may suggest that readers of *The Arthritis Cure* who find themselves reading *Arthritis Begone!* would not appear to have found the ultimate answer to their problems in the earlier book. I hope and believe that there is an excellent chance that it is here.

My own first encounters with the miseries of arthritis began when I was in my forties and enjoying a life that was modestly active. The first symptom, which seemed unaccountable then, but which I now know is often a precursor of arthritis, was spontaneous low back strain for which there was no apparent external cause. Seeking a consult with an orthopedic surgeon, I underwent the obligatory examination including X-rays. "Can't find anything wrong!" the orthopedist said, trying to sound reassuring. Then I developed right shoulder pain, followed some months later by severe pain, tenderness and swelling in my right wrist. These later events, like the low back strain, left no clues detectable on the X-rays.

This time, I took my troubles to an internist, another specialist who deals frequently with arthritis. He examined me carefully and concluded that I had a rotator cuff strain in my shoulder and tendinitis in my wrist as the result, he said, of my piano-playing. I couldn't help observing privately that piano-playing is a two-handed activity; by the internist's logic, I ought to have troublesome symptoms on the left side as well, which was not the case. Still, I was relieved to hear that my colleague thought something other than hypochondria was the cause of my troubles; this time, it appeared, some circumstance traceable to my body was not quite right. My internist prescribed ibuprofen, a nonsteroidal anti-inflammatory drug or NSAID, as a palliative, but it relieved neither the underlying inflammation nor the pain. On my own, I decided to try some crude experiments with my diet, beginning with the amounts of caffeine and alcohol I was consuming. When I cut back on either one for a number of days, I began to feel somewhat better. I mentioned this coincidence to my doctors, but orthopedist and internist alike dismissed it as irrelevant.

The tendinitis eventually receded, but then about twelve years ago I developed new troubles. Severe pains settled into my back, hips, knees and neck. Ordinary movement became difficult. This time there seemed to be no doubt. X-rays and blood tests both confirmed arthritis, specifically osteoarthritis. (This is the most common form of arthritis. Mainstream rheumatologists consider it to be an age-related result of the breakdown of cartilage that normally acts as a cushioning between bones: they often describe it as ''degenerative arthritis.'')

This time my rheumatologist prescribed Naprosyn, a more potent NSAID, to ease the discomfort. He told me I should be satisfied if treatment kept my arthritis from getting any worse. Reversal and cure, he indicated, was rather unlikely. Discouraging words, indeed. Worse yet, the new drug, like the analgesic before it, gave me only slight relief at best.

Desperate to free myself of what was fast becoming unbearably severe pain, I began to review in my mind the experiences of some of my patients on hormone therapy. I wondered if their therapeutic retreat from arthritis symptoms might not have relevance for me. Being a physician, and consequently able to prescribe medications for myself outside the usual guidelines, I decided to experiment using my own body as the test case. Almost immediately after I began taking small doses of replacement estrogen and progesterone, I experienced mild pain relief and greater freedom of movement, but not enough for reasonable comfort. This led me to extend my experiment to related hormones, and I next tried spironolactone, a progesterone derivative conventionally prescribed to reduce high blood pressure and fluid retention, or edema.

Within 24 hours of beginning the regimen of spironolactone, I experienced dramatic relief from pain and stiffness. Better yet, this pain relief grew over the next two to three months until my symptoms had all but disappeared. Somehow, through a novel pairing of dietary changes and unconventional drugs, I had helped myself to a new lease on life!

With my newfound confidence, and wanting to know whether my experience was a fluke or if it was something that could relieve other similarly afflicted people, I tried the same treatment on several gynecological patients in my practice and on male friends who were also severely troubled with arthritis. Many, but not all of them, experienced relief comparable to my own reaction. Armed with these findings, I tried to interest other physicians in the community in extending the experimental work informally. No one stepped forward.

I then went to the University of Connecticut in Farmington, where I was a clinical associate in the Department of Obstetrics and Gynecology. I invited my Ob-Gyn colleagues to involve themselves in further studies, on the grounds that arthritis was a frequent complaint within the population of older women we served. With scarcely any debate, the department turned me down. Next, I contacted my peers in the University's Department of Rheumatology, offering to share data with them in the hopes that they would carry forward what I had begun. The rheumatologists also turned me down, claiming that they had neither the time nor the money for unconventional approaches. I also approached the federal government's National Institutes of Health in Bethesda, Maryland, where an army of researchers is supposed to be spearheading investigations into new and better medical treatments. They, too, declined to look at my evidence for "lack of time and money."

All these turndowns might have discouraged a more practical man, but I was neither particularly surprised nor shaken in my resolve. The medical profession is well-known for its territoriality—practitioners offering suggestions from outside the professorial fraternity are often rejected outright, and even those within the medical fraternity who propose heretical notions have a hard time being taken seriously. Yet I knew with absolute certainty that I was onto something very, very important; it deserved attention, whatever the obstacles. Consequently, I continued over the next few years to refine my hormonal treatments, first as part of my private practice, with the full knowledge and cooperation of over 300 of my own patients, and later, through collaborative research with another like-minded scientist.

I would now like to share with you the story about one of my patients that exemplifies the hard-nosed resistance by the medical establishment, even when a "miracle" was submitted to their continuing care. The patient, whom I will call Oliver V #1, was a 68-year-old partly disabled World War II veteran, who had become a successful farmer. Oliver had developed three severe problems: progressively worsening osteoarthritis of 20 years' duration; dozens of open, never-healing, painful sores all over his body for twelve years; and muscular weakness and areas of numbness for several years. The Veterans Administration had been unable to dent his arthritis with NSAIDs and cortisone shots. His painful sores did not respond at all to any measure of their therapies including medicated dressings, antibiotics, psychotherapy and skin grafting which involved weeks of hospitalization. The sores, which varied up to 4 by 2 inches in size, and which excavated down to his muscles in depth, gained the official diagnosis of a "psychosomatic manifestation"! Nothing was offered for his weakness and numbness.

My beginning therapy was with vitamins C and E in megadosage along with EPA, or fish oil. With the new system of Microdose prednisone (I'll explain about that shortly), I made his arthritis 94 percent better. Then I started shots of vitamin B12 every three days. Within three days all pain, swelling and redness of the sores were gone! Within two weeks, as if by incredible magic, all lesions were covered by skin or scab, including the four-inch lesion!! The muscular weakness and numbness were gone! He was a new man—again an able farmer.

The Veterans Administration Hospital and doctors now refuse to supply these proven-to-be-effective medications to which this war-disabled veteran is entitled, because they deem it to be "nonsense"! Oliver must now buy his own entitled medication in order to remain in good health. Our governmental system was agreeable to paying countless thousands of dollars on a standard, 100 percent losing battle, but not one penny on a proven but unconventional 98 percent victory! They might well take care of him again if only he would return with his initially disabling arthritis, sores and weakness! Incredible?

In 1991, my arthritis work had its first major breakthrough. That year I met Professor Virgil Stenberg, Ph.D., Department of Chemistry, at the University of North Dakota at Grand Forks. Stenberg, as it turned out, was also conducting independent experiments in treating rheumatoid arthritis, and for reasons not unlike mine. Dr. Stenberg's wife, Helen, had suffered from severe rheumatoid arthritis for many years, and he had come to realize that medical science fell short when it came to controlling the pain, swelling and bony disfigurements she endured. Stenberg, believing that he might be able to help her and to contribute something to the medical field at the same time, began by studying the underlying nature of inflammation. Like all good scientific experimenters in human health, he started with laboratory rats as his research models.

Over the course of 12 years, Stenberg determined that prednisone, a corticosteroid drug with a multitude of therapeutic uses, could help to compensate for the body's loss of natural corticosteroid hormones, a deficit characteristic of arthritis. Prednisone would reliably reduce the rat inflammation. Stenberg devised his theory of cyclic prednisone administration, called Microdose, which, when administered to Helen, brought about excellent and persisting relief of her arthritis.

Dr. Stenberg also had ideas regarding foods and their role in allergic reaction in arthritis. Through a process of trial and error, he was eventually able to isolate wheat as a trigger of his wife's arthritis flare-ups. Once wheat was eliminated from her diet, she gained near-normal freedom from arthritis pain and stiffness. Stenberg's next step was to support his findings through a double-blind pilot study of approximately 30 patients, which he carried out with the cooperation of physicians at the University of North Dakota Medical School. Once again, his results were remarkable, outperforming any other system of treatment known at that time.

After lengthy personal discussions, Dr. Stenberg and I decided to put our systems together in an innovative program for arthritis treatment. To support our work, we established a nonprofit research facility in Grand Forks which we called the Inflammation Institute. The idea was to create a demonstration clinic where we could prove to both patients and physicians that our methods offered an improvement over those of conventional rheumatology in terms of efficacy, safety and cost. Hundreds of patients who came from all over the United States thought our work was miraculous, but never did even one doctor avail himself of our advertised free information and training.

Over the next 14 months nearly 500 patients came to the Institute for treatment. Almost all of them did so after becoming discouraged by the poor results of the conventional rheumatological care they had received elsewhere. By contrast, using the combined therapies developed by Dr. Stenberg and myself, these same patients experienced, on average, a diminution of their arthritis symptoms by about 70 to 75 percent. Indeed, several of our patients were able to dispense with the canes, walkers and even wheelchairs they came in with. And some, who had come to us fully expecting that they would have to go through the knee and hip replacement surgeries their previous physicians had recommended, found that the surgeries were no longer necessary.

One Native American patient, who had been medically certified as totally and permanently disabled, and who was anticipating spending the rest of her life in a long-term care facility, experienced 75 percent symptomatic improvement by our methods, and then went to college. As news of our success spread, patients came from further and further away, until we could fairly say that every rheumatologist in the State of North Dakota had "contributed" two or more dramatically responding patients to our care. Patients from all over the United States and Canada also began to hear about our work and appear for evaluation and treatment. The equilibrium of the physicians of the State of North Dakota was so upset by my miraculous results that they arranged to remove my state license to practice medicine!

As mentioned earlier, my approach to arthritis control and treatment is not only less expensive and more effective, but it is extremely safe. Standard therapy for arthritis is almost entirely focused on pain relief through the common over-the-counter remedies—analgesics such as aspirin and acetaminophen, if they work, and various NSAIDs, including ibuprofen and naproxen (Naprosyn), if something stronger is indicated. Such drugs, while only mildly toxic in small doses over the short term, may have dangerous cumulative effects when taken over many weeks and months, as is often the case in serious arthritis management. Together, NSAIDs have been implicated in 10,000 to 20,000 deaths from stomach ulceration, hemorrhage or perforation annually in the United States (Roan, 1996). The NSAIDs are also responsible for 15 percent of the kidney damage that eventually requires renal dialysis in the U.S. (Pernager et al. 1994).

At the Inflammation Institute, I did not prescribe even aspirin for anyone. And under our system of medications, no serious side effects have been experienced, nor are they anticipated. Over a period of nearly twenty years, none of our combined therapies has even remotely threatened any patient's life. Quite the contrary, in fact; our hormone replacement therapy goes beyond arthritis relief to actually increase life expectancy in that it coincidentally inhibits bone loss (osteoporosis) and arteriosclerosis (narrowing of arteries that can lead to heart attack and stroke) which are common accompaniments to the aging process.

Reduced cost is another benefit of my approach to arthritis treatment. The cost of following the regimen recommended by the Inflammation Institute varied from $15 to $1,000 per year, depending upon the kind and combination of drugs deemed appropriate for the individual case. By contrast, the average rheumatic patient spends $3,000 annually on medications and therapy to treat the same condition. Add to these diminished expenses the savings in canceled joint replacement surgery and in the return of once-disabled wage-earners to the work force, and my economic argument becomes even more persuasive.

My motivation in writing this book is to share with the many millions of arthritis sufferers who live in this country and abroad the knowledge and relief I have gained through my investigations. The number of people who can gain from this advice is staggering. According to the Centers for Disease Control, the current figure of 38 million arthritis sufferers will swell to 44 million by the year 2000. I believe that at least ten million of these individuals can be made more comfortable merely through adoption of my Food Elimination Diet, described in detail in Chapter 4, entitled "Food and Arthritis: The Odd Coupling." And they can do it at no cost other than the small price of this book. Many millions more, whose arthritis is triggered by other circumstances, could gain markedly improved health with the cooperation of their doctors, were they to take up the full range of recommendations I offer.

In the chapters that follow, I will additionally inform you about my basic concepts concerning the biological development of arthritis in your body, so that you can better understand your disease. I will also tell you in greater detail about effective, safe and relatively inexpensive treatment approaches, including medications for arthritis. Some of these are vitamin supplements, available on the open shelves of your pharmacy or health food store; others are prescription drugs, available only with the cooperation of your doctor who must write the orders. Buy a second copy of this book for your doctor so that he can also read and understand what you have learned. If any doubts or questions should remain after reading this book, I encourage readers to write to me at the location given at the end of the book.

Should you feel awkwardness in pressing your doctor into doing that which you are convinced has merit, remember that it is reasonable for you to be proactive in your own health care. If your doctor will not listen, find another doctor who will work with you. Just as you do not spend your hard-earned money for clothing that you don't like or that does not fit you, shop for your doctor carefully until you find one who fits.

By now you will have recognized that among physicians, my view of the doctor/patient relationship is somewhat unconventional. I specifically reject the traditional notion that your physician alone should mastermind the management of your illness. I feel strongly that the patient needs to be fundamentally engaged in the critical choices surrounding his or her care. Whether you like it or not, you as a patient "own" your disease. Consequently, your motivation to heal exceeds that of all other people offering advice and treatment.

In my experience, patients who are encouraged to be actively involved in their own care can also contribute very good observations regarding the causes of their medical problems. Certainly, the patient's sensitivity to his or her symptoms is greater than anyone else's. By listening carefully to what my patients tell me, and translating the information into medical terms, I can invariably make more progress more quickly toward finding them relief than if I act autonomously on their behalf.

This is not to say, of course, that you can proceed without any physician support. Physicians hold the keys to a great storehouse of medical knowledge that can be indispensable in guiding and evaluating your progress. To procure a physician who will work with you to obtain the best possible care, without spending a fortune for obtaining nothing, I will tell you what I tell my patients:

1. Get the names of the doctors who treat arthritis in your area. When I say "area," you should understand that we are talking about a geographical region that may be many miles across, requiring some travel on your part to find a suitable physician. A doctor who has no ears to hear is of zero value to you!

2. Upon making your first exploratory telephone appointment, tell the nurse or receptionist the specific purpose of your visit and confirm the appointment only after being assured that the doctor is at least open to such give-and-take of information.

3. Carefully explain at the very beginning of the visit, and before there is any examination, that you want the doctor to give serious consideration to continuing the medications you have already found to be effective and without side effects, and to work with the treatment systems outlined in this book. Be prepared to supply your doctor with a copy of this book so that he or she can carefully read and study exactly what you are requesting.

4. If the doctor refuses to comply with your prestated request as negotiated with the nurse, terminate the visit immediately, before he performs any billable service. And do not be persuaded by his arguments to accept substitutions for the procedures described here, because all alternatives are likely to be more dangerous, more costly and less effective. Do not pay for a nothing visit.

5. When you find a cooperative doctor, please quickly spread his or her name to your hurting friends.

The basic purpose of this book is to supply information about recent advances in arthritis theory and therapy to arthritis patients and physicians alike. I have made my explanations simple enough to allow people not trained in medical science to understand, yet technical enough to convince scientists that the theoretical concepts are reasonable and valid. It is possible that this will be the most rewarding learning you will ever experience in terms of gaining physical comfort for the rest of your life. If any part of this book should prove difficult reading for you, you can pick up on the simplified summations in the sections labeled REMEMBER that appear at the end of each chapter. In addition, the summary at the conclusion of the book presents a synthesis of the basic concepts for your review once again.

In the 1540s the Italian anatomist Vesalius said that the heart worked like a pump. Within the academic world of his day, he and his ideas were widely scorned. Seventy-five years later, William Harvey said essentially the same thing, and his observations launched a revolution in medical science! Perhaps someday the ideas on arthritis causation and treatment presented here will likewise be viewed as the incontrovertible truths I believe them to be.

2

Some Basic Features of Arthritis

ONE DISEASE WITH MANY FACES

BEFORE WE get into the specifics of arthritis treatment in subsequent chapters, let me familiarize you with both the vocabulary and some of my basic theories regarding arthritis and arthritis management. I must warn you that some of my theories diverge sharply from those held by most modern rheumatologists. Since my system of therapy has been working so much better than traditional treatments, it would suggest that I am onto something very important and that you can benefit from what I have to teach. In this chapter I start out to organize the hodgepodge of existing information about arthritis into a very workable hypothetical system, to which I have added some new details of my own. You will learn that there is only one disease of arthritis that comes in different forms determined genetically, that the problem arises mostly from a faultily performing immune system that cannot handle all the trouble it produces, and that ideal therapy entails removal of the causative factors and bolstering the natural defenses against inflammation.

The information that follows must of necessity be somewhat technical and detailed if you are to understand why I treat arthritis as I do. Ideally, you will learn from it to "be your own doctor" by adapting these ideas to your own circumstances and symptoms, rather than accepting in blind faith the standard treatments that are traditionally meted out. It is not mandatory that you understand or remember everything that is contained here, but to insure that you get the essentials, I include brief summaries at the end of each section. Those of you who are curious about details may digest all of the paragraphs, while those of you who want just a rough idea can snack on the summaries. The more you become familiarized with the many bits of information, the more the subject matter will mean to you, and the greater the likelihood that you will find relief from pain. And so, get ready to go to work on your own behalf! In this chapter you will find out that all forms of arthritis, no matter by what names you know them, are basically the same disease caused by the inability of your immune system to cope with an overabundance of immune complexes.

How Many Rheumatic Diseases Are There?

Rheumatologists identify over 100 different rheumatic diseases and approach treatment as though each of the diseases had a different set of causes and effects. I, on the other hand, approach arthritis as a single disease of irritation/inflammation. You may call it osteoarthritis (degeneration of joint cartilage), fibromyalgia, rheumatoid arthritis, lupus or gout, but I believe that each and every case can be traced to a common cause. I treat them all according to the same basic principles.

Arthritis literally means "inflammation of the joints." The term is often modified by the additional description "rheumatoid," which is derived from a Greek term meaning "flowing or moving back and forth from place to place." Rheumatoid arthritis is pain in your joints that comes and goes and can travel from one joint to another. Arthritis may even erupt outside the joints as in fibromyalgia, where the arthritis attacks your muscles; in scleroderma, where it stiffens your skin; or in lupus where it may be associated with destruction of your kidneys.

Arthritis affects far more females than males; and, while it affects people of all ages, including babies, it most commonly makes its first appearance in the decade between ages 50 and 60. According to the American Academy of Orthopedic Surgeons, osteoarthritis is the leading cause of disability in people over 55, and few older persons escape it entirely.

The onset of arthritis varies from gradual to sudden; but, once it arrives, it rarely goes away completely. The painful inflammation of the joints may lead to their gradual destruction and ultimately to surgical joint replacement. The inflammation of nerves may lead to numbness and paralysis. Though most cases are no worse than partially disabling, there are uncommon instances in which the patient's heart or kidneys are so damaged as to shorten life.

The factors that trigger arthritis remain a matter of lively debate, with viruses, bacteria, physical trauma, psychological factors and malfunction of the immune system all having their proponents. The immune system is designed to attack and destroy alien invaders, such as bacteria. Many authorities have concluded that arthritis is an autoimmune disease, which means that the immune system attacks and destroys the joints of afflicted individuals. The tendency for the immune system to make mistakes in identification of your own body tissues is an inheritable feature; and, once a mistake has been made, there is a tendency for further misidentifications.

Medical science up to now has been very nearly powerless to satisfactorily overcome the relentless, painful incursions of rheumatic disease. There is no recognized cure for rheumatic disease, and the conventional therapies to date have very little success to boast about. Even the standard medications, which are widely prescribed and used, are thought by many physicians to have so many side effects as to be of questionable value.

HEREDITY'S ROLE

It is widely accepted, whatever the precipitating cause of arthritis might be, that heredity plays an important role not only in susceptibility, but also in the type of arthritis you display when it appears. Heredity is the process by which the characteristics of body and temperament are passed from the biological parents to the child as part of reproduction. Each individual is composed of heritable material contributed equally by the sperm and egg. The function and development of each cell of your being is controlled or programmed by a capsule within that cell called a nucleus. The nucleus contains 23 different pairs of structures called chromosomes. In turn, each of these chromosomes consists of a long strand of DNA material which is arranged in lines of almost countless small hereditary units called genes. It is estimated that there are about 500,000 genes altogether in the nucleus. The structure and consecutive arrangements of genes vary subtly from person to person, which accounts for the infinite variety that we find in the human family, from the color of your eyes and hair to your susceptibility to arthritis. The genetic makeup of certain groups of people with similar diseases has been found to be very similar, and that is expressed as Human Lymphocyte Antigen, such as HLA B-27 for arthritis and HLA B-4 for diabetes. It is believed that small subgroups of HLA genes determine the type or pattern of arthritis (*e.g.* lupus, gout) that is manifested in any one person.

One aspect of the body that tends to show family patterns is the programming of your hypothalamus, a small, central part of your brain that regulates many basic functions of your body. Most particularly, the hypothalamus management of cortisol, which controls your arthritis inflammation, seems to be inherited. If either or both parents carry the genes that result in less-than-optimum delivery of cortisol, there is a good possibility that you too have a predisposition for this problem. The tendency may vary from strong to weak, but the chances are good that some viral or bacterial disease, or even a severe fracture, will eventually produce sufficient hypothalamic stress to allow your rheumatic disease to erupt.

The specific pattern of rheumatic disease which the predisposed body demonstrates, such as rheumatoid arthritis, lupus or osteoarthritis is also established genetically. All the patients in a group investigated by E. Szanto et al. (1983), who developed low back arthritis after a severe pelvic infection, were found to be of a specific hereditary tissue type, HLA B-27, while those patients without that tissue type did not develop the arthritis even though they had the identical pelvic infection. In sum, if you have arthritis, its development was determined in large measure by the genetic cards you were dealt at conception, and in a smaller measure by the stress events in your life.

The Immune System's Role

The immune response is an intricate biochemical system of defenses designed to protect your body from materials that are recognized as foreign, or "antigenic." The usual antigens are viruses and bacteria, but an antigen can be any chemical structure from foods to environmental chemicals to hormones that may be perceived by your immune system to be alien.

Some antigens are made of two separate parts that become antigenic only when they combine. One part of such an antigen combination is called the basic protein or, as I prefer to call it, the potential antigenic protein. That potential antigenic protein all by itself is never a problem. But when it combines with its partner, which we call a hapten, the hapten can make the pair reactive. If one were to replace the "bad guy" hapten of this antigen pair with another very, very similar, yet only slightly different "good guy" hapten, the resultant combination would no longer be looked upon as an alien by the immune system. Accordingly, one of the principal goals of the arthritis therapy I describe is finding ways to substitute nonreactive, slightly different haptens for those that trigger antigenic reactions, and thereby turn off the mechanism that is producing your inflammatory pain.

In arthritis, the hapten that triggers the antigenic response is usually a hormone that has been produced by the body itself with the intent of performing important functions of metabolism. Some "fault" in the function of the immune system causes it to mistake that hormone, in combination with its carrier protein, for an alien substance. It is not known why the immune system goes awry to work against its own tissues and hormones. All we can propose at present is that the immune system "misreads" the information it receives and reacts according to the mistaken perception that the body is under attack. The result, of course, is warfare on a cellular or biochemical level.

The principal soldiers in carrying out the surveillance and attacking foreign invaders are the white blood cells, or more formally, "leukocytes," which travel through the bloodstream in the company of red cells and platelets. There are many millions of white blood cells, of several different subtypes, in circulation. They provide multiple layers of protection, first by chemically attacking, and then engulfing and digesting, unwanted substances in the body.

The most numerous white cells are the polymorphonuclear leukocytes, familiarly called "polys," and they spearhead the fight at the site of injury, surrounding and digesting bacteria and other small particles in a process called phagocytosis, literally "eating by cells." Another subtype, accounting for roughly one in four of the white blood cells, are the lymphocytes, which are further differentiated as B cells and T cells. B cells produce the freely circulating proteins known as antibodies, that bind themselves to antigens, interfere with the antigen action and make them more visible to other defenders. T cells also make antibody, but they carry their antibodies on their surfaces. It usually takes several days for the lymphocytes to learn how to make a new antibody to a new antigen, and that is why most of our minor illnesses get better in about a week. Usually that defensive ability to make a specific antibody is never forgotten by the lymphocytes, but, for some viral infections, the memory may be only of short duration.

The antibodies made by the lymphocytes are also known as immunoglobulins, and play a central role in the immune responses triggered by allergies and hypersensitivity reactions. Since T lymphocytes carry their immunoglobulins, or antibodies, on their cell surface, so their action is called cellular immunity.

The next group of white cells of the immune system is called monocytes while circulating in the blood. The monocytes are believed to transform themselves into macrophages (large eaters). Special concentrations of macrophages are found in the liver, spleen, lymph nodes and bone marrow as well as in points of inflammation. They have the ability to wander about the body to wherever they are needed. They ingest and digest old cellular debris, including worn out red blood cells and abnormal cancer cells. Importantly, they in-

gest and process antigen so that it may be presented to the lymphocytes in such a way that the lymphocytes can learn to structure
antibodies specifically against that antigen.

Disposal of Immune Complexes

When antigen and antibody combine, they form an immune complex.
The immune complexes are of two basic types: one in which a reproducing infectious agent is present as the antigen, and the second
wherein a non-reproducing chemical such as a food or a hormone
is present as the antigen. In both situations, the immune system is
programmed to eat up and digest the antigen, but in the case of the
bacteria some of them may be resistant to the efforts of the
macrophage.

In rheumatic disease, the inflammation occurs when one of two
possible things goes wrong and the immune system is unable to cope:
either so many immune complexes are made that the phagocytes
cannot possibly eat them all up, or the phagocytes lose some of their
ability to eat and destroy even a normal number of complexes. Either
of the two problems results in excess immune complexes freely circulating in the blood. The excess immune complexes filter out of the
bloodstream to collect in the tissues at various predetermined locations. There they meet up and react with a chemical system called
complement which is a normal constituent of the blood and is made
up of twelve protein particles. The reaction with complement produces
a large number of inflammatory chemicals, resulting in swelling, redness,
heat and pain, and an abundance of irritating chemicals, causing numbness, weakness, paralysis, pain and altered bone growth. In summary,
unless the phagocytes are able to eliminate the immune complexes ex-
peditiously, irritation/inflammation are threatened.

Your immune system forms the primary defense against inflammation by eating up immune complexes, while the secondary
defense against inflammation is managed by your hypothalamus
which creates a burst of cortisol for control of the inflammation

produced by the immune complexes that escape the primary defense and filter into joints. See Figure 2-1.

IMMUNITY VS. ALLERGY

Immunity is a protective system that is designed to cope with the constant invasion of dangerous agents so that they cannot do long-term damage to the body. We cannot survive without our immune system being intact, as is clearly demonstrated in the deadly consequences of AIDS, which robs individuals of their normal defenses against infectious agents and cancer.

By contrast, an allergy is an excessive, inappropriate, explosive form of immunity. It tends to arise most frequently as the result of exposure of the skin to a chemical, of the respiratory system to particles of pollen or dust, or of the stomach or intestines to a particular food which, in the majority of people, causes no such reaction.

Sometimes it is unclear in a patient whether a certain reaction is due to immunity or allergy. We can, for example, find an inhalant such as tobacco causing both asthma and rheumatic disease, and menstrual hormones causing both rheumatic disease and asthma. There are three standard, related sensitivity conditions that tend to occur in the same patient: rheumatic disease, irritable bowel syndrome and asthma. The basic principles are the same: when an alien substance is introduced, the body learns to make a chemical defense. When the same adverse chemical is again introduced at a later time, the body may display a strong adverse reaction and perhaps an inability to deal with the large quantity of reactive factors or complexes produced.

The ideal way to handle any form of immune reactivity is to detect the offending antigen and then eliminate it from the reactive patient. This can be accomplished by not eating offending foods, by controlling chronic mycoplasma infection, and by inhibiting the production of natural hormones which have become reactive with the immune system.

When the antigen cannot practically be removed, we must bolster the defenses. This may be accomplished by supplying extra-large

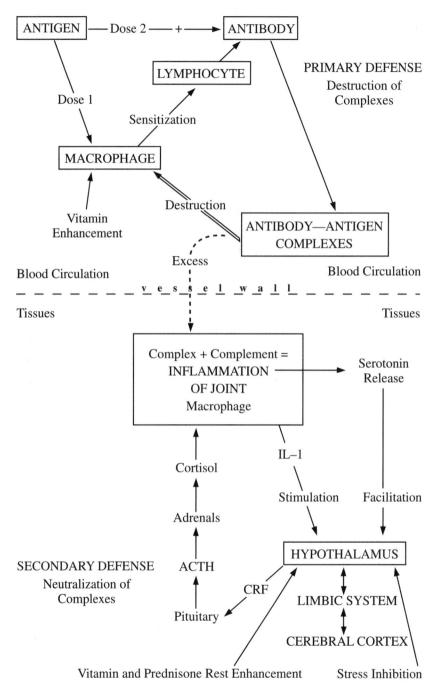

Figure 2-1. The Two Inflammation Defense Systems

amounts of the required metabolic materials (vitamins) to nourish and enable the phagocytes, and/or by using prednisone to compensate for inadequate hypothalamic cortisol responses to inflammation (to be described in detail in Chapter 8).

Another method favored by some physicians is desensitization, or immunotherapy, in which the patient is given gradually increasing doses of the allergen until the immune system becomes less reactive in some rather obscure manner. Though good results have been reported, my experience relative to arthritis is that the shots and drops are of essentially no benefit. The difference in beneficial response for skin and respiratory problems possibly lies in the mechanisms of globulin G in immunity-arthritis versus globulin E in allergy-asthma.

Occasionally individuals will develop what are called multiple chemical sensitivities, which make them highly sensitive, chiefly via the nose, to environmental stimulants. Common agents are insecticides, solvents, auto emissions and cigarettes. Once the first sensitization has been developed by a major exposure, subsequent sensitivities appear more easily. Response to the chemicals may produce emotional and psychiatric disturbances, and occasionally joints will become arthritically inflamed.

INTERACTION OF YOUR BRAIN AND DISEASE

Even though we do not fully understand the complexities of the brain, evidence is accumulating that there are distinct and important interactions between the conscious and subconscious psyche, and further, that those coordinated functions may be altered by immune reactions and chemical sensitivities. Your conscious thoughts are managed by your large cerebral cortex while your subconscious thoughts are governed by the smaller hypothalamus-limbus portion of your brain. Research has shown that immune reactions can be diminished or turned off through suggestive hypnosis and by the power of positive thinking for wellness. Psychosis, mania and depression have often been found to be caused by contact with internal and external immune chemical factors. I am certain beyond doubt the tension of the premenstrual syndrome (PMS) is an expression of autoimmunity. Some medical institutions are now investigating the effectiveness of hypnotic suggestion for the control of rheumatic disease and cancer, both of which are related to deficient function of the immune system.

CONVENTIONAL WISDOM ON RHEUMATIC DISEASE

At this point I must introduce to you the standard, modern theory of the cause of rheumatic disease. I tell you not because I believe it to be true, but because I think it is wrong, and because I think that in its wrongness lie the reasons that modern treatment of the disease has been so unsatisfactory.

Although physicians are divided as to whether rheumatic disease is uniformly an autoimmune disease going on in the joints, they do agree that rheumatoid arthritis, a commonly severe type, has autoimmunity at its core. But they also believe that since the disease is generated by antibodies to joint tissue antigen, there is no practical way to intervene in and eliminate the process. The best hope they offer with their therapies is to modify or partly counteract the antibody-antigen reaction, which involves *suppressing* the functioning of the body's defense against inimical intruders, the immune system. By the end of this book I hope that I will have persuaded you of this old concept's invalidity and of the fundamental logic of my own new approach, including *enhancement* of immune function.

GYNECIC TISSUES

Women are particularly prone to rheumatic disease, with two out of three of those suffering from it being women, and also to painful disturbances of menstruation. Through my research I have found that the internal sexual organs and tissues produce a potential antigenic protein which may combine with an ovarian hapten progesterone to form important antigenic complexes. I use the term *gynecic* to refer to those female tissues as a group. I have found that under certain circumstances the best way to stop the formation of reactive hormonal immune complexes, and thereby relieve immune disease arthritis as well as some associated immune neurological diseases, is surgical removal of the gynecic tissues. I go into this subject in detail in Appendix A.

STEROIDS

Nowadays the word steroid tends to have a number of unpleasant, even unhealthy, connotations. This is because of reports in the news media that steroids are sometimes used improperly by athletes to enhance strength and muscular development, and that such misuse can have very dangerous physical and psychological after-effects. There are also widely publicized reports of very serious side-effects resulting from the use of high doses of cortisone for the treatment of rheumatic disease. But when steroids are used knowledgeably and properly in the treatment of rheumatic disease, they can be extremely beneficial.

Cholesterol is an important constituent of body cells, essential for producing new cells and certain hormones. Manufactured by the liver, it is also taken into the body in a wide variety of foods in our diet. Genetics play an important role in determining how much of your ordinary diet is converted into cholesterol. The basic chemical structure of cholesterol is that of a steroid, so you eat steroids every day.

Alterations in the structure of this basic cholesterol structure are made by various enzyme systems. With each small change in structure, a different steroid is created with different functions in regulating the body. In this way we make within ourselves such steroid sex hormones as estrogen, progesterone and testosterone, and such adrenal hormones as cortisol and aldosterone. You can see the amazingly close structural relationships between several of these steroids in Figure 6-1 in Chapter 6.

Biochemists in their laboratories have learned to create chemical structures that have many similarities to natural steroids. And pharmaceutical scientists have found ingenious ways to turn the chemical structures into medications, often of a specificity that gives them advantages over the natural originals. Examples of some of these man-made steroids are: prednisone to replace cortisol; the progestins norgestrel, norethindrone, ethynodiol diacetate and medroxyprogesterone acetate to replace progesterone; and mestranol and ethinyl estradiol to replace estrogen. A drug called spironolactone (discussed in Chapter 9), a restructured version of the steroid progesterone, has unique powers for altering steroid production and function in ways that may help relieve your arthritis.

My hope is that the steroid chemists of the future will be able to create still more of these alternative preparations so that they may be able to do the job even more effectively and also that they will be available in case the immune system should learn to react adversely to the presently available medical formulations.

Normally the body's glands produce steroids at a rate that keeps the system humming nicely, with neither too much nor too little of any one substance circulating. As the demand for hormones is constantly fluctuating, the body also has natural monitors designed to regulate production. If a given hormone is in ample supply for the tasks on hand, the sensors take note of that and tell the gland to slow production; this process is called feedback inhibition. Then, for example, if cortisol is replaced by an ample supply of look-alike prednisone, the adrenals by a process of feedback inhibition will halt their production of cortisol. A similar feedback inhibition may occur relative to the ovaries and adrenal glands when native antigenic progesterone is replaced by nonantigenic progestins. The potential antigenic hapten progesterone may thereby be put out of production by the progestin feedback, and the rheumatic activity would be halted.

BLOCKING OR COMPETITIVE BINDING

In order for hormones to exert their influence upon tissue metabolism, they must become attached or bound to the cell over which they are to exert their control. This occurs in a manner that can be compared to a key fitting into a lock, the hormone having a particular shape (key) and the cell surface having an equally specific receptor site (lock), and the two molecular shapes engaging with precision. Usually the hormones are accompanied to their work site, which may be distant from their point of manufacture, by carrier proteins to which they have become just lightly bound. When they get to their destination, the light protein carrier binding is relinquished in favor of the competitively stronger cellular receptor's attraction. One form of therapy which I describe in greater detail in later chapters is to send in competitive medications that block the attachment of the inflammation-causing antigens before they have a chance to start the damaging rheumatic process.

REPLACEMENT THERAPY

When the controls become damaged, and hormone supplies are no longer what they should be, a variety of illnesses large and small are likely to occur. It then becomes the role of the physician to heal the damaged controls or to adjust the hormones by replacement medications.

DIAGNOSING YOUR ARTHRITIS

How can you, a layman, determine that you have arthritis? The principles that I will teach you are really so amazingly simple that you will have no difficulty in being your own diagnostician. If you want the same diagnosis done accurately by your rheumatologist, be prepared to leave about $1,000 with him.

We all injure ourselves with cuts, strains and broken bones. Part of the initial healing process is inflammation, which causes pain. With younger people healing occurs rather swiftly; but, as we get older, the healing takes longer and longer. For some of us older, arthritic folk, the pain never seems to go away after injury. The common patterns of complete healing are six weeks for a cut, bruise or strain and six months following a major bone break and resetting. If the pain lasts longer than these ample limits, it becomes reasonable to assume that arthritis is involved. Persistent pain indicates that full healing of the inflammation has failed.

The various pain problems that may arise from ordinary exercising, such as tennis, golf or raking leaves may result in such conditions as tendinitis, tenosynovitis, sciatica, bursitis, tennis elbow and water on the knee. These represent the beginnings of arthritis, as do "causeless" strains of your neck and shoulders. If the pain and discomfort do not go away in six weeks, you might want to look for relief using the arthritis measures outlined in this book. If they cause so little discomfort that you can live with them for now, keep this book where you can find it later, because you can bet on the symptoms becoming more severe in the years to come.

The lower back is a very common place for rheumatic aches and pains. The frequency of backache is particularly high in older people. Low backaches are variously attributed to lumbago, sciatica, bad posture, bad sleeping habits, slipped disc, heavy lifting, sacroiliitis, and only infrequently to the real answer of arthritis. The problem for doctors making the specific diagnosis of arthritis in the early stages is that the condition rarely shows up in X-rays and other laboratory tests. This leads many physicians to suspect the patient of malingering or having a psychological rather than a physical problem. My basic diagnostic tool is your account of persistent pain.

Can you be wrong in your diagnosis? Yes, it could always be a cancer or an infection, but I have never seen one. If you are in doubt about your safety, spend a wad of dough with your doctor to alleviate your fears. Then when he says there is nothing wrong, but it still hurts too much, give my arthritis program a try. For many of you, you will start to feel better within two weeks. That's how long it takes to discover that you can moderate pain and inflammation by something so simple as eliminating one or more common foods from your diet.

REMEMBER

1. Though arthritis expresses itself in many forms, it is nonetheless a single disease of irritation/inflammation.
2. Your particular form of arthritis (osteo, rheumatoid, etc.) is determined in large part by heredity, over which you have no control.
3. At the root of all arthritis is an error in the immune system, which is designed to protect the body from germ invaders, but which

occasionally misperceives other chemicals as the enemy (antigen) and launches an immune attack.

4. There are three sources of antigens: hormones, foods and infectious agents.

5. The immune system attacks antigens in two stages, producing antibodies to neutralize them by forming immune complexes, and subsequently launching phagocytes to eat up the complexes.

6. Allergies are similar in nature to autoimmune responses, but tend to occur from touch and airborne chemicals.

7. The rheumatic disease state arises when the immune system's fighters are unable to keep up with the production of immune complexes, the excess of which spills over into the joints and other tissues to create inflammation. The greater the spill-over, the greater the inflammation.

8. Native hormones in the body and the steroids engineered in the laboratory are critical elements both in causing and treating rheumatic disease.

9. Replacement hormones, with little or no antigenic effect of their own, may beat out antigenic native hormones for position on the target cells. In so doing, they may successfully ward off the rheumatic response.

3
Know Your Enemy

KEEPING YOUR DAILY PAIN SCORE

AN OUTSTANDING problem in rheumatology has been how to establish accurately not only whether inflammation is present, but also how to reliably determine the degree to which that inflammation changes under the influence of therapy. It has been conventional for rheumatologists to determine this by physical examination for the count of tender and swollen joints. This is very time-consuming and costly. This approach, in going by the evidence of just one particular day and time, also fails to take into account how much your condition may vary from day to day and week to week. And it is of limited value in monitoring those patients whose pains exist without detectable tenderness or swelling in the joints.

Clearly, you and your physician need a better system, so in this chapter I offer you one by which you can easily and accurately measure and monitor how much arthritis pain you have on a daily basis. If you are a little bit better today, you will now have a way to express just how much better. If you want to compare the hurt you feel today with how much you hurt a week ago or six months ago, you will now be able to make that distinction.

I came to this system after many years of struggling unproductively with the problem of measuring patient pain. I knew that having a reliable method of determining how the total pain my patients experienced changed from one visit to the next was the key to assessing the value of my therapy. Then I had the good fortune to work with Dr. Stenberg in North Dakota. Stenberg was in the process of developing such a system, and working together, we further refined its particulars to better meet the needs of accuracy and simplicity. With still more recent revisions, what I call the Daily Pain Score monitoring system was born.

The Daily Pain Score charts some 40 joints and groups of joints in your body. Accompanying it is a Daily Pain Score Guide which provides a series of numbers from zero to nine by which to convert the subjective language of your pain experience to something more objective and quantifiable. To chart your daily pain, you must consider each joint listed, enter the appropriate number in the column provided, and add them up to obtain your total pain and inflammation score for that day. Since rheumatic disease pain is well known to vary from day to day, you must keep score for a week and then average the seven total pain scores to establish your Baseline (or beginning) Total Pain Score.

You can see how it works in the sample Pain Score Chart (Figure 3-1). The chart forms and the Pain Score Guide appear in Appendix D.

When there is considerable fluctuation of your Daily Total Pain Score, I tend to think of food reactivity as the cause, though that is not always true.

The system may seem a little complicated at first, but after you have used it for just a few days, I think you will find it very easy indeed. It takes no more than a few minutes at the start of each day to fill in the chart which is printed at the end of this book, and you will be able to keep good track of your progress. Though it is not absolutely perfect, it is a very long step forward in making a difficult job much easier. Be sure to photocopy the chart, both front and back, before you make any entries. The simplest record to keep will be with front and back on one piece of paper and will represent the numbered days for an entire month on just one paper. It might be more convenient to copy your Pain Score Guide as well.

DAILY PAIN SCORE: Name: _____ Month: _____

Day of the month			1	2	3	4	5	6	7	8	9	10	11	12	13	14	15	16
Jaw																		
Neck																		
Chest																		
Low Back																		
Hip		L																
		R																
Knee		L																
		R																
Ankle		L																
		R																
Foot	Heel	L																
		R																
	Front	L																
		R																
Shoulder		L																
		R																
Elbow		L																
		R																
Wrist		L																
		R																
Thumb	Base	L																
		R																
	Mid	L																
		R																
Pointer	Base	L																
		R																
	Mid	L																
		R																
Third	Base	L																
		R																
	Mid	L																
		R																
Ring	Base	L																
		R																
	Mid	L																
		R																
Little	Base	L																
		R																
	Mid	L																
		R																
Total Pain Score																		
Prednisone																		
Spironolactone																		
Progestin																		
Antibiotic																		
FED and others																		

Notes:

Figure 3-1. Daily Pain Score.

This simple measure of evaluation has been measured to be at least equal to a physician's examination for accuracy, and superior to it for sensitivity. And you can imagine how expensive a daily physician exam would be!

Once you have established a baseline number, you are ready to begin the therapeutic measures recommended elsewhere in this book. This is because you need a beginning baseline reference point for evaluating any changes that may occur. You need to know where you have come from to appreciate how far you will be going towards relief from arthritis pain.

Incidentally, don't be too concerned if you can't find the descriptive word and number in the Pain Score Guide that properly expresses your feeling. If you consistently apply a number that is a little higher or lower than the next person in keeping his or her score, it doesn't matter very much, because what you are looking for is relative changes, and these will become apparent over time, however you assign numbers. The most important feature of the total pain score is not how large or small it might be, but how much it changes in response to a measure of therapy. Whether your score changes from 100 to 50 or from 10 to 5, the improvement is still 50 percent and the measure of therapy has to be regarded as significantly effective. By the same token, if your score goes down five points from 100 to 95, those five points have less meaning than going from 10 to 5.

It is important for you to do the scoring at the same time each day, preferably in the morning a little while after arising from bed. Scores taken later in the day may be either higher or lower, so they can only be compared to other later-in-the-day scores. Morning is generally the best time, especially when you are using prednisone, discussed in Chapter 8, because you should decide right then whether you need to take that morning medication that day or not. Morning is also the time when stressed muscles have had an entire night to recover on their own, if they will, during bed rest. For those people who work during the nights and sleep during the day, the same principle of scoring on awakening still applies.

Save the running record of your Daily Pain Scores in your personal home medical file from the very beginning—it can be of great importance. A factual record makes up for faulty memories. Take, as an example, the experience of a patient whom I will call Bob A

#2. Bob, who suffered from osteoarthritis, started with a baseline total pain score of 100.

After he began taking his prednisone, his score dropped rapidly to 25, and he felt as though he had been reborn. Several months later, however, Bob began to complain to me that more severe pain was returning. He asked if I could come up with some new medication to make him as comfortable as he had been at the time of his first big, wonderful drop. But when I took a closer look at his Daily Pain Score, I found that it was down to 12, half the score that he had in an earlier time deemed miraculous! Bob scratched his head in utter amazement, but I recognized a common phenomenon at work: When we are first relieved of a very large amount of pain, it really feels so-o-o *good* that whatever remains seems minor indeed. But, as the months pass and our threshold of tolerance changes, we are more easily bothered by even low levels of residual pain. Having lost track of where we came from, we naturally become dissatisfied again. Even though the Daily Pain Score showed that Bob had actually continued to improve since his first big prednisone-induced drop, he had convinced himself that the medicine was becoming ineffective. Having the Daily Pain Score to fall back upon was invaluable in revealing the tricks played by Mother Nature upon him and his memory.

It is very important to record even the slightest pain in any of your joints so as to get a complete picture of the disease's progress and actions, so don't be tempted to play down any sensations you honestly feel. Even if the pain is genuinely slight, give it the low number it deserves, because the information may reveal important clues that you or your physician would otherwise miss.

To see how true this is, imagine a patient who comes in complaining of a sore knee. I take down the information, but I tell him I want him to pay equal attention to all his joints. This patient protests that it is only the right knee that he cares about, not all the other stuff. I explain why I want the details as follows: Let us suppose that his baseline score is 27, to which his right knee is found to contribute a factor of 7. I then prescribe medication and in one month he returns with a total pain score that has fallen to 7. When we examine the pain chart, we find that all of the remaining 7 points are now localized in his right knee. Had we not done the total scoring, he might claim that in as much as his right knee had not changed, the medicine was no good at all and that we should find a better one. However, the Daily Pain Score reveals that his medication is working very well, effectively ridding him of most of his symptoms. As a result, we do not look for a replacement medicine; rather, he continues to take the medicine as before and I order an X-ray and a surgical consultation, on the theory that the knee problem may be traceable to bone fragments, to a tumor or to a microbial infection, any of which will need therapy particular to it.

Or consider this example: Suppose you start with fifteen joints hurting to which you assign values of 3 points each for a total pain score of 45. After one month of therapy you report that you are getting worse, that one joint now is routinely scoring 6, and that you want me to come up with a new approach. However, your Daily Pain Score analysis reveals that your total pain score is now down to a mere 15, with three joints rated at 3, one joint at 6, and the remaining eleven joints having no pain at all. As your physician, I tell you that you have improved 66 percent overall, thanks to the medicine you are taking and that you should be more patient; that other improvements will almost certainly come in time.

What do I do to combat the remaining pain? I now *add*, rather than replace, successive measures of therapy step by step to bring the score down still further. Each therapy that improves the total pain score becomes a permanent part of your daily regimen. Any therapy that fails to deliver any measure of relief, as charted in the total pain score, is deemed not effective and should be discarded.

I make it a point not to start more than one therapeutic measure at a time, and I do not start another until the previous one has been fully evaluated, because it is important to detect how much change is made in the baseline score with each new therapy. This approach, as you can see, is remarkably simple, one that you yourself can easily judge and manage.

USING THE DAILY PAIN SCORE

As I mentioned, a copy of your Daily Pain Score chart is located at the back of this book. I recommend that you get at least a dozen photocopies made of both sides, using one for each month of the year.

Note that there is an entry at the bottom of the Daily Pain Score for each of the four most common medications you might be taking—prednisone, spironolactone, progestin and any of the antibiotics. Use an X in the daily space to denote the standard dose, except with prednisone and tetracycline, for which you should record the specific number of pills taken daily. You will find another line to track abstinence from a certain food or some other food regimen you may be following, again using the X. Vitamin B12 is important in my treatment program, as I'll discuss in Chapter 4, so be sure to mark down every B12 shot taken, too, and informally note any other factors such as stress, an infection, or physical injury, that could conceivably be related to your arthritis experience.

There may be occasions when it is appropriate to do an additional pain score at a time of day other than the morning, for example when you experience a major rapid flare-up of pain caused by some such adverse factor as a reaction-producing food. When using prednisone, this identification of a flare could justify immediate medication to prevent a surge of inflammation from getting further out of control. Do not alter the initial pain score entered for the day, but enter the new total pain score, the time, and the dose of prednisone in the space below that day.

A few helpful afterthoughts: If your pain is mostly in your muscles, as in fibromyalgia, decide which joints the pains are closer to and record the pains in those joint spaces on the chart. One specific joint which has almost no pain at rest would initially merit a score of no more than 2, but in action it earns a score of 6. To resolve the disparate rest-action numbers, average them as 4, which is to be entered for the day. Since the majority of your joints usually will have a score of zero, just let the blank spaces represent zero. A pocket calculator may help you in adding long columns of numbers as well as determining your average baseline scores.

This system of number recording has allowed me to make rapid and accurate telephone evaluations for patients up to 10,000 miles away. The record usually speaks louder than words.

With the aid of such daily evaluations, you are now in a position to detect how your body responds to the myriad factors that affect your arthritis—foods, medicines, menstruation, minor and major illnesses, emotional stresses and the weather. You can now participate in your own treatment. This is not to suggest, of course, that you go it alone completely. You must continue to rely upon your friendly and knowledgeable doctor for annual checkups, advice and the safe monitoring of your prescription medicines. But with this approach, and by following the therapies discussed further on, you can comfortably award yourself, as I do my patients at the end of their training period, the honorary degree of "Doctor of Your Own Arthritis."

REMEMBER

1. Your quick and easy pain scoring is equal to or better than the accuracy of your doctor's daily examination.
2. Success for therapy is measured by the change of your pain score rather than how high it can be.
3. Your pain score may detect a toxic factor in your environment.
4. Your pain score is a lasting, reliable record of how you feel.

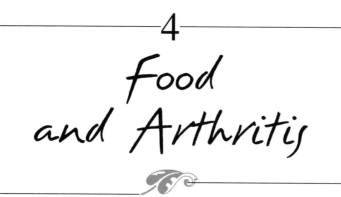

4
Food and Arthritis

THE ODD COUPLING

GOOD HEALTH includes feeling well and performing well. Appropriate nutrition—chiefly supplied by the food we eat—provides the raw materials for maintaining that good health. To get there and stay there, we need to know on an individual basis not only what we should eat but which foods are better avoided because of systemic reactions, sometimes subtle, that the culprits may cause. In this chapter, we will explore the relationship between foods and their production of rheumatic disease, discuss some of the specifics relating to individual reactions to certain foods, and finally describe how you can sort out and eliminate your own "bad news foods" so as to reduce or even end your own arthritis pain.

FOOD AS RAW MATERIALS

Let's begin with some basics regarding the role of food in general. Your body needs at least 40 different chemical constituents, from calcium to zinc, to keep in good running order. With the exception of a few chemicals that you breathe in the air, and some others that you take in water or with the help of sunlight, they all come from the natural constituents of food. Most of them are provided in the form of complex compounds that have been broken down and reassembled to fulfill the body's needs. The process of breakdown and reconstruction, known as metabolism, begins almost immediately after the foods enter your mouth. Chewing breaks up solid foods into more manageable bits, and saliva adds enzymes that further contribute to dissolving the compounds.

As the materials pass through the various chambers of the digestive system, they continue to be transformed until they are liquefied and in a condition to be absorbed into the intestinal walls. From there the chemical nutrients are ultimately transported via the blood and lymph capillaries throughout the body where they are put to work building new bone, muscle and blood, replacing and replenishing cells that are worn out or damaged, providing heat and energy, and conducting myriad electrochemical processes such as the transmission of nerve signals from the brain to the furthest extremities in the fingers and toes.

Nutrients are divided according to their chemical composition and their biological roles into three main groups of macronutrients: carbohydrates, proteins and fats, along with a number of essential vitamins and minerals. Some chemical combinations can be created by our internal cellular laboratories if the laboratories are supplied with the necessary components, but many vital chemicals are beyond our body's manufacturing capabilities; they must therefore be supplied in finished form from outside sources, chiefly foods. Among these chemicals are vital amines, popularly known as vitamins.

Though no one can yet say what a perfect diet is, we do know that a good diet supplies you with adequate amounts of each and every one of the chemical components essential to life. For people who suffer from disorders involving chemical imbalances, determining a healthful diet becomes a more difficult issue, but, as I describe later in this chapter, it can be addressed successfully if everyone involved is willing to approach the question with a degree of patience and an open mind.

Let me first say that I am not aware of any food or group of foods that will specifically protect you from getting arthritis or relieve the arthritis inflammation you already have. Nor do I know of any ordinary food that will significantly enhance the twin engines of conventional arthritis relief: phagocytosis, the process by which certain specialized white cells gobble up and destroy bacteria, immune complexes and other waste materials in the system; and the production of cortisol, the naturally-occurring steroid hormone that counters tissues' tendency to swell when irritated.

On the other hand, I do know that there are certain foods that may trigger arthritis flare-ups in susceptible individuals, and it is here that I believe you can take an active role in treating yourself. The foundation of my therapeutic system is what I call the Arthritis Food Elimination Diet, and in the pages that follow, I will tell you how to zero in on the specific agents that may be causing your arthritic reactions. If one or more foods do turn out to play a role in your arthritis, and you can identify them by name, you then have the relatively easy task of eliminating them from your diet.

HOW REACTIVE FOODS WORK

Food can be a powerful force among the three basic agents responsible for rheumatic disease. The food or foods may produce pain and swelling symptoms indirectly through the workings of the immune system which has an immune reaction to them. At other times, foods are in effect co-conspirators, giving an extra measure of potency to the pains produced by the two other reactive factors in the pain of between 25 and 28 percent of all the patients I see for arthritis treatment. I base this upon the fact that, through identifying and then removing specific foods from their diets, all of these patients have improved significantly.

Though the prestigious Arthritis Foundation has rejected this premise, there are a handful of scientists today who concur with me. One of these is rheumatologist Richard Panusch, M.D. (1986), who has published excellent clinical investigations that support the relationship between certain foods and rheumatic disease. Another is Marshall Mandell, M.D., past medical director of the New England Foundation for Allergic and Environmental Diseases and a bioecologist, whose book *Dr. Mandell's 5-Day Allergy Relief System* (1988) clearly demonstrates a food connection for allergies in general. Dr. Mandell's book, by extension, suggests that this allergic reaction relates to the immune reactivity that takes place in arthritis. (Like me, Dr. Mandell has found the medical establishment resistant to his unconventional findings, despite the quality of his research and the impressive record of his therapy.) Van de Laar (1992 a,b) clearly supports the arthritis food viewpoint.

Here, in a nutshell, is the chemical basis of food reactivity as an agent in rheumatoid arthritis, as it is currently understood. After the chemical constituents of your food have been absorbed into your blood and lymph, and are in the process of being transported to the various organs, tissues and cells that will use them, they are under constant surveillance by the cells of your immune system. The role of the immune system, of course, is to screen for harmful, usually infectious, agents and to destroy them before they have a chance to multiply and overwhelm the body.

For reasons unknown, the immune system can occasionally make big mistakes in some people, turning immune cells against some body hormones, or incorrectly recognizing once-welcome nutrients as toxic substances. When this happens, the immune system becomes the agent of immune disease, causing among several painful events a degree of heat, swelling and inflammation. Worse yet, once that error has been established, it becomes part of the immune system's permanent program; consequently, all further encounters with the misidentified substance produce the same dire response. Since we do not as yet know how to correct the faulty immune programming, it becomes our task in treating various forms of arthritis to learn how to circumvent that programming.

There are three general patterns of reactivity to foods. The first can be called a *fixed allergy,* in that the specific immune response is a permanent, unchanging, adverse reaction to a food, no matter how frequently or infrequently it is encountered.

The second is a *cyclic allergy,* in which the degree of symptomatic response is diminished very markedly if a sufficient interval of time is allowed to pass between encounters with the causative food. The usual cycle time is five to seven days. In this cyclic allergy, it seems that between encounters the immune system is capable of forgetting just how much it despised the foe. But the forgetting is only partial, and should the reactive person eat the same food again the next day, the immune system will have regrouped,   resulting in a significant arthritis reaction.

Lastly, there is the *addictive allergy*, which may produce some symptoms while the food is in the body, and even stronger reactions when it is withdrawn. Coffee is a familiar example of the addictive allergen. It is common to experience a headache that appears when coffee has not been consumed for a certain number of hours, and goes away within a few minutes of taking a new cup of coffee.

Complicating this picture is the fact that arthritis can also be caused by immunity to one or more of the steroid hormones that are made by your own body. This is called autoimmunity or allergy to oneself. It is important to understand that the symptoms of arthritis triggered in this manner cannot be distinguished from those caused by food reactivity. This is demonstrated by the experience of a 68-year-old woman suffering from rheumatoid arthritis. Lucy J #3 came to me with a baseline total pain score of 117, high by any standard. Over a period of time and through trial and error, I found that she was reactive to a combination of food (wheat) and autoimmune factors (natural hormones). When I assisted her in eliminating the wheat and controlling the natural hormones, her pain score went down to zero! When either factor was reintroduced, her pain rose substantially—to 40 with the wheat and to 90 with the hormone. The pain was expressed in virtually identical joint locations, though with different intensities. This told me that in her case the pain of rheumatoid arthritis was essentially a summation of the two factors. If both a food substance and a hormone antigen produce in effect the same disease complex in a patient, either separately or in combination, it becomes reasonable to presume that each factor is capable of activating the identical mechanism for the production of that disease. From this it follows that any corrective therapy must address both issues if the inflammatory process is to be brought under complete control.

My experience with patients indicates that the reactive foods implicated in rheumatoid arthritis are almost exclusively of the fixed, unchanging type. This differs somewhat from Dr. Mandell's cyclic findings on reactions to food among a broad spectrum of respiratory tract patients. The difference possibly lies in the involvement of immunoglobulin G in arthritis and immunoglobulin E in the respiratory patients. I am cautious about using the cyclic approach to food elimination in the case of arthritis, because I worry that the repeated introduction of antigens risks exacerbating the immune system's underlying general responsiveness. Easier and more gratifying in the long run for most people, I believe, is a diet that avoids challenging the immune system altogether once the reactive food or foods are identified. If, on the other hand, you are reactive to such a very large number of foods that your basic nutrition is jeopardized, then I would recommend adopting a rotation system that allows for eating each of the cyclic foods in sequence, say one each day on a five- to seven-day rotation. Though I keep looking for it, I have never encountered a cyclic food allergy response in my arthritis patients.

To demonstrate further how diverse food reactivity can manifest itself as an agent in arthritis, let me cite another case, that of Betty M #4. Betty, aged 60, was diagnosed as having osteoarthritis eight years before I saw her. She had been prescribed NSAIDs, which proved to be of little or no help in treating the pain and were very hard on her stomach. She was then switched to a course of daily oral prednisone, but it afforded only temporary relief. When Betty first came to see me, we established her baseline total pain score to be 55, and then she began the food elimination diet. By charting the changes in her pain, we soon narrowed the allergic reaction down to oranges, grapefruit and tomatoes. Once she eliminated these trouble foods from her diet, her pain plummeted to 6, and during the next five months her pain score was further reduced to a mere 1 or 2. When she experiences a rare, small flare-up of arthritis pain, the use of Microdose prednisone eliminates the problem.

Not everyone responds as dramatically, but the average relief of pain in the 25 percent of patients who respond to this approach is about 50 percent. Other treatments are used in the hope of decreasing the residual pain. It surely makes sense to test yourself, and if you discover a food or foods that provoke an arthritic reaction, you will be at least a partial winner for life. The Food Elimination Diet is totally safe and it costs you nothing to carry it out.

THE FOOD ELIMINATION DIET

The Food Elimination Diet (FED) is designed to help you identify and remove from your diet only those foods which cause *your* arthritis. Other physicians offer other concepts of dietary arthritis control—the Dong Diet, the nightshade diet, the rotation diet, et cetera. The problem with the other diets is that they are fixed, and there is no one diet that will reliably conquer the problem for all. It is always worthwhile following the FED to arrive at a diet custom-made for you.

The FED is not a totally new concept, but uses the strong points of several diets. Identification of reactive foods is done through trial and error in four successive steps.

STEP ONE: BASELINE TOTAL PAIN SCORE

The first step in your dietary investigation is to familiarize yourself with the total pain score and to establish your baseline total pain score while you are using your normal variety of foods. The baseline result will give you something to measure against as you later tinker with your diet. All progress is relative. If your pain score starts at 50 and comes down to 20 in response to the diet, you can consider yourself a winner. If you achieve no pain relief at all, you have at least learned that food is not a causative agent for you and that you must look elsewhere for improved health and comfort.

STEP TWO: CLASS I DIET

In this second step of your investigation, I want you to look at the following Table of Food Classification (also reproduced in Appendix C, where its location makes photocopying easier—put one on your refrigerator door for easy daily reference).

The top row of Class I foods is what constitutes your *investigating diet,* which will last at least seven days. Class I is made up of a number of fruits, vegetables, starches, oils and fish, which statistically have the least possibility for a reaction. While this is admittedly limited in choices, it is well balanced, and if you had to, you could live indefinitely on this class alone. Of course it is possible that even these simple foods may cause you, as an individual, reactive problems. If you already suspect that to be the case with any item, do

TABLE OF FOOD CLASSIFICATIONS
FOR FOOD ELIMINATION DIET

Fruits	Vegetables	Sugar-Starch	Oils	Meat	Other
CLASS 1. EASY FOODS FOR YOUR BASIC DIET:					
Grape	Lettuce	Rice	Olive	Fish plain	Ample water
Peach	Avocado			Cod	Salt as
Pear	Celery			Flounder	needed
Plum	Olives			Salmon	
Prune	Parsley-flakes			Tuna	
	Cauliflower			*OR* Turkey	
	Peas				
	Spinach				
	Winter squash				
CLASS 2. O.K. FOODS FOR 48 HOUR ADD-ON ONE BY ONE:					
Apricot	Asparagus	Honey	Canola	Catfish	Carob
Blueberry	Cucumber	Maple Syrup	Safflower	Herring	White
Cantaloupe	Eggplant	Sugar		Trout	vinegar
Cherry	Onion	Tapioca			
Pineapple	Rutabaga				
Rhubarb	Summer squash				
Watermelon	Sweet potato				
CLASS 3. BE CAREFUL—FOODS FOR 48 HOUR ADD-ON:					
Apple	Beet	Brown sugar	Sunflower	Chicken	Non-caffeine
Banana	Broccoli	Kidney Beans		Lamb	soda
Cranberry	Cabbage	Lentils		Venison	Herbal teas
Coconut	Garlic	Lima beans			
Dates	Kale	Navy beans			
Figs	Mushroom				
	Swiss chard				
CLASS 4. BE VERY CAREFUL—FOODS FOR 48 HOUR ADD-ON:					
Tangerine	Carrot	Barley	Margarine	Anchovy	Cinnamon
	Peppers	Almond	from soy	Clam	Mustard
	White potato	Cashew	(Parkay	Scallop	Vanilla
		Pecan	light)	Oyster	Spices— pepper
		Walnut			M-S-Glutamate
CLASS 5. *BEWARE*—FOODS FOR 48 HOUR ADD-ON:					
Grapefruit	Corn	Oats	Corn oil	Beef	Milk
Lemon		Rye	margarine	Pork	Cheese
Lime		Wheat	(no	Crab	creamed
Orange		Peanuts	whey)	Lobster	cultured
Strawberry		Yeast	Peanut oil	Shrimp	Yogurt, whey
Tomato					Eggs
					Chocolate
					Coffee
					Colas
					Tea
					Alcohol

READ ALL FOOD LABELS CAREFULLY

not eat it during this testing process. Do not eat anything that you do not see listed in class I.

As you read the foods of Class I, you will see turkey listed as an alternative to fish as a source of protein. Use turkey only if you know you are reactive to fish; otherwise, fish is to be preferred because it has a smaller likelihood of causing a reaction than turkey. Bake, boil, poach or fry the fish. You may eat canned tuna, but only the water-packed variety. Use olive oil for frying the fish, for "buttering" your vegetables and rice, and as a salad dressing. Canned fruit also fits here, but only when prepared in its own natural juices; cans marked "in syrup" contain various sugars and are to be avoided for now. Limit your food seasonings to parsley and salt. Check the label on the brand of salt you use to be sure it does not contain even micro-amounts of corn sugar, an additive sometimes used instead of calcium silicate to promote easy pouring. No lemon on the fish at this stage of the test! Remember, the pleasure promised with this diet was never intended to be in terms of gustatory satisfaction, but from the relief of arthritic symptoms—a relief which, with a little luck, you may experience with the greatest of joy!

Do not jeopardize the test results by starting your diet test during a holiday season, when social eating engagements will surely get in your way. Once you start the diet, you must *not* eat or drink anything whatsoever (other than water) that you do not see in the Class I listing until the initial testing time is completed. DO take all the routine arthritis medicines you are currently taking; otherwise you will not know if changes are due to diet change or medication changes. If you should feel so well that you no longer need the medicines—and many patients have achieved this wonderful result— you can try stopping them gradually after the initial testing phase is over.

I give the following case report to demonstrate not only that the diet can be very rewarding for pain relief, but also that you can maintain vigorous health almost indefinitely on these few foods. Walter P #5, a 55-year-old farmer, called in March 1992 to report that his life was "going down the tubes" because of his severe arthritis, which a local specialist had diagnosed as ankylosing spondylitis, a painful and eventually immobilizing inflammation of the vertebrae. The disease had come on relentlessly, Walter reported, and in a matter

of a few years he found himself barely able to walk; he was consequently unable to work his farm. In financial straits as a result, he
said he could not pay me unless I made him well enough to resume
farming. Seeing how great his predicament was, I agreed to his all-
or-nothing proposition.

The first measure of therapy I instituted was to have Walter find
his baseline total pain score, which turned out to be 56. Next, I put
him on the FED, starting as always with the Class I diet. By the end
of the first week, Walter's pain score was starting to drop; and, by
the end of three weeks, he was recording an astonishing 3 total! In
fact, he came to feel so well over the months that followed that he
was able within a short time to return to active farming. Beginning
that spring, he planted his usual acreage of crops, and was able to
harvest them in the fall. He found that he was even able to run
around his fields, literally, to do his chores and to drive, maintain
and repair his huge farming machines.

During all that time, I could not persuade Walter to go beyond
Class I foods. His experience with ankylosing spondylitis had so
traumatized him that he dared not experiment with unknown foods
when he had something that was working so well. Though he lost
ten pounds in the beginning, Walter's weight soon leveled off, and
he began to regain his normal strength and vigor. Only after the
harvest was in did he resume his investigations with the rest of the
FED. Coffee was eventually isolated as his major problem. Walter
was more than able to pay his bill, and did so with gratitude.

The pattern of Walter's pain scores—a large drop almost immediately, followed by continued but less dramatic improvements in the
weeks following—is seen often with caffeine. It can take five full days
or more for the last traces of some reactive foods to leave your body.
By the end of seven days you will have a reliable clue from your
accumulated scores as to whether the diet is helping or not. If you find
no favorable change in your pain scores by then, it means that foods
do not play an influential role in triggering your arthritis. You can then
discontinue the diet altogether, or go on to the Draconian methods described in the section on fasting several pages later. If, on the other
hand, you do see improvement, you have discovered something very
important, and you should go on to Step Three, below.

Occasionally patients complain, after having been on the Class I
diet for only two or three days, that they feel weak, dizzy, headachy
and even more pained. Their feelings are no doubt genuine. But I can

assure you that the causes are not to be found in the paucity of foods allowed in the diet. Rather, they arise from such factors as chemical withdrawal from one or more withdrawal-reactive foods and from psychological factors we all feel from denying ourselves favorite foods. Whatever the reason, I strongly recommend that you not quit prematurely. Remember the phrase "no pain, no gain." Your ultimate reward for staying the course would be very great, if you emerge from the experience having thrown off the shackles of debilitating arthritis.

In talking about the psychological resistance to eliminating favorite foods that some patients exhibit, I am reminded of George F #6. George was a short, feisty, 70-year-old who arrived at my office bent over and walking with difficulty from his osteoarthritis. Once seated, he was scarcely able to get out of his chair to be examined because of stiffness and pain. To begin my treatment of his condition, I had George first take a week to work up his pain score, after which I put him on Class I FED. By the third day of the FED, his score was down by half. George decided to celebrate his progress, and he ate a piece of banana nut bread. His score promptly went back up to where it started. His subsequent course of spironolactone was of no value. A course of prednisone made only mild inroads into his discomfort. When I urged George to resume his FED investigations, telling him that I thought we were on the verge of finding that he had an allergic reaction to wheat, he refused to continue. He loudly informed me, as he once again needed help to get out of his chair, that he would be damned if he would give up his daily doughnut and coffee with his buddies at the coffee shop. I thought that I had seen the last of this single-minded fellow, but about nine months later George returned to my office for a continuing supply of prednisone. I was amazed to see that he was now standing straight, and that he was able to sit down and stand up easily. When I inquired as to what miracle had brought this good change about, he explained that he had finally been forced to realize that he preferred pain relief to his beloved wheat snack after all. I did refill George's prescription, but with the primary arthritis triggerer removed, he found he needed prednisone only occasionally and in very low doses to remove minor aches and pains.

STEP THREE: ADDING BACK FOODS

Once you've completed the Class I diet, and established a new and lower baseline for pain, you're definitely on the right track. Not only do you have reasonable evidence that food is at least part of your arthritis problem, but also you have a reliable yardstick against which to test other foods for allergenic properties. You still don't know, however, which of the many foods on the chart constitute the enemy. In order to make that identification, selectively and systematically add to the initial Class I diet the foods belonging to Classes II through V.

You can, should you prefer, choose foods for trial from any of these groups in any sequence you like. But, generally speaking, the best way is to work your way in order from the lower-numbered classes to the higher. The reason is that I have assigned each food to its particular class based upon the potential I know it to have for causing an arthritis reaction. Thus, your chances for avoiding a problem with a Class II or Class III food (broccoli or chicken) are substantially better than are your chances of tolerating a Class IV or V food (wheat or caffeine). So, if you leave the most likely candidates for trouble until last, you will be eating a more varied diet of agreeable foods sooner than if you leapfrog immediately to some of the statistically more allergenic foods and then suffer a set-back that slows you down. On the other hand, you may argue that the higher-numbered foods tend to be more pleasing to your taste, and you want gratification now. Either way works. It is really just a matter of personal choice.

When you are adding a new food to your diet, take it in unusually large amounts for two consecutive days, so that if you do have a reaction, it will be dramatic enough to detect and measure easily. If you have an allergic reaction, it usually occurs in just a few hours, but it certainly will occur within 24 to 48 hours, and with a reaction you can rapidly progress from feeling limber and pain-free to being stiff, in considerable pain, or even incapacitated or bedridden. Cyclic sensitivities will not become apparent until the repeat exposure on the second day, but we still consider that the reaction began within the first 24 hours because the underlying causes were kicked into gear then.

Following any measurable pain response to a food, you must wait for however many days it takes to get back to your baseline pain score before moving on to the next food. You cannot detect a reactive food if your pain score is already up! By testing from the baseline, you will always get a fair and impartial reading of each food as you take it, whereas as long as your score remains elevated by a reactive food, detection of the second food is impossible. As each new food is tested and found to be nonreactive, add it to your basic list of Class I foods, to be eaten whenever you please. Ultimately your diet will consist of all ordinary foods except those few that you have ruled out because of pain reactions.

When adding foods, watch out for compound foods such as bread, soups, sauces and alcoholic beverages, which are composed of multiple ingredients. Before you add bread to your diet, for example, you need to test not only how well you tolerate wheat or other relevant grains, but also how reactive your system is to milk, eggs, yeast and so on, each one individually. Margarines are another compound food, with almost all of them containing not only one or more vegetable oils but also milk whey; Parkay light is one of the few that do not. Read the labels of prepared foods, which by definition are compound foods. Corn products are among the most widely used additives in prepared foods—as thickeners, sweeteners, cooking oils as well as vegetables—and must be tested for individual reactivity before you consume them in any combination. Cornstarch can even creep into certain brands of table salt, where it is used to keep the moisture-absorbing grains flowing freely.

Notice that I have placed at the very bottom of the Class V foods one highly popular food—coffee and its essential ingredient, the stimulant caffeine. Coffee is, in my experience, *the* food most likely to cause arthritis reactions. Even in arthritis-free patients I have found caffeine to be the most frequent source of unpleasant symptoms, including stomach acid, bleeding ulcers, abdominal pains, bloody diarrhea, rectal and vaginal irritations, breast tenderness and lumps, chest pains, bladder irritability, insomnia, emotional irritability . . . and the list goes on. And this bearer of so many troubles is not limited to the stimulating hot drink that so many enjoy. Caffeine is also a stimulant occurring naturally in tea, cocoa and chocolate products, and in kola nuts, the last-named being an element of cola carbonated drinks. Caffeine is also added to some pain medications (Excedrin for one) and even remains in measurable quantities in products labeled decaffeinated (the caffeine is in fact, only partly removed). As I noted earlier, coffee and caffeine fall into the uncommon third category of addictive allergens. Their adverse withdrawal effects may be relieved within a very few minutes of consuming the chemical, as in the rapid cessation of a caffeine-withdrawal headache upon drinking a cup of coffee, but the negative rheumatic effects will continue. Coffee reactivity may be almost imperceptibly gradual and cumulative from day to day, though sometimes it may be strong and rapid. Coffee sensitivity is not restricted to its caffeine alone, but may be due to a combination of the many other potentially reactive chemicals found in the coffee bean.

And at least during the FED testing period, avoid if you possibly can eating restaurant and fast foods, whose ingredients are known for sure only to their chefs. The most effective dietary control is managed by you, in your own home, your own lunch pail and your own picnic basket.

When you have finished the first round of testing all the foods you would like to eat, return to take a closer look at each of the foods you suspect caused a reaction. I suggest that you test each one separately twice more before drumming them out forever, because it is always possible that some other unconnected event, such as a spontaneous rheumatic flare-up from menstrual hormones, caused the numbers to rise. Observe once again whether the foods cause a reaction on the first day for a fixed reactivity or on the second day for a cyclic reactivity, on the chance that you might still be able to eat the food intermittently and in moderation. Leave caffeine to the very end for testing, because it takes up to three weeks to raise a pain reaction and perhaps another three weeks to rid the body of its effects, all of which demands considerable patience to test properly.

STEP FOUR: MAINTENANCE

Ultimately, you will arrive at a diet custom-made for you. This puts your diet leagues ahead of all the other one-size-fits-all diets offered as curatives for arthritis patients. I urge you to stay on your custom diet forever, since fixed sensitivities nearly never go away. I urge you not to have ''holidays'' for taking the ''forbidden fruits,'' because I feel that is coaxing the immune system to become more angry.

TOUGHER INVESTIGATIVE STANDARDS FOR SOME

The Food Elimination Diet described above is neither difficult nor, regrettably, perfect as a system for detecting food allergens in all individuals. This imperfection is due to the fact that you could be one of the less than 5 percent of the population who have an allergy to one of the low-reactive foods included in the Class I diet, where initial testing usually begins. Much as I might wish it so, not even the fish, rice and olive oil are universally safe for every single living individual.

How do we do the FED for these people? The only answer for the tiny minority for whom the standard FED fails to detect a possible problem is to consider total fasting for five days to see if the total pain score will now drop down. If the pain does decrease, then you will introduce each of the Class I foods one at a time. During the five-day fast, drink at least three quarts of plain water every day to maintain healthful fluid levels. Stop the use of any and all tobacco products if you use them, and take a dose of milk of magnesia to remove any residual chemicals from your digestive system that might compromise test results. Also avoid any pills, including vitamins, minerals, aspirin and prescription drugs that are not essential. If in doubt about the safety of stopping your current medications, discuss the matter with your physician, telling him why first. The reason to avoid the pills is that almost every medication you take contains potentially reactive binding agents, such as starch, lactose, sucrose, gelatin, cellulose, shellac and various dyes to give the pill physical strength, shape, color and taste. Almost every NSAID available contains a form of starch. The larger the pills and the greater the number taken, the more likely they are to interfere with the FED. A dozen aspirin tablets a day could make a sizable difference, while one methotrexate tablet per week might be undetectable.

I did not include this restriction of medications, particularly NSAIDs, in introducing the Class I diet, but I now suggest it for those who did not obtain satisfactory relief on the low-reactive diet and who still harbor a suspicion that some food is a contributing factor. This is because the withdrawal of painkillers at this juncture is almost certain to result in a temporary increase in the level of pain, and that would discourage many faint-hearted patients from undertaking the valuable basic, 95 percent effective, diet investigation at all. The fast is used by some who want a complete investigation the first time around. Should you choose to proceed in this manner, stop taking your NSAID two or three days before the fast to get a measure on what your natural baseline score would be.

During the five days of fasting, expect to lose five or more pounds of body weight, and as much as 20 pounds if your body is retaining large quantities of fluids due to edema. Also expect to feel very hungry for the first two days, and then to have those hunger sensations diminish later. Some people report increased physical pain and weakness, and emotional irritability in the first few days. Such reactions are transient and represent a withdrawal reaction to a reactive food that is being eliminated—actually good! Further along in the fast you may even notice that your mind and body are truly becoming stronger and more comfortable. (One of my young arthritis patients, when I first saw her, had been totally disabled mentally, as evidenced by her inability to concentrate long enough to finish a sentence. During the diet, as her pain score diminished, she became mentally focused for the first time in years. She subsequently went on to become rehabilitated in every sense when she identified and eliminated caffeine from her diet.) Bowel irritations, headaches, asthma, heart pains and so on, may possibly go away during your diet time. Be sure to tabulate each and every one of your reactions/ changes as they occur daily so that you can later make accurate comparisons with your new status on the FED.

Most patients, when I describe the five-day water fast, react in horror. But I can assure you that, unless you have some other unrelated medical condition that makes fasting unhealthy, you can do it without seriously compromising your ability to carry out the rest of your daily activities. I speak from personal experience. In the Korean War I was one of several hundred heavily laden soldiers to hike five days over mountains with nothing more than water from the streams to fill our stomachs. We suffered neither headaches, faintness nor weakness, but we did become skinnier in the process. In recent years I again did the five-day fast without problems.

If at the end of your five-day fast, your pain score has made a significant drop, then you start introducing Class I foods one by one at two-day intervals. Do the same with your medications. Then you should proceed similarly with the rest of the foods on the chart.

At some point you may read about some kind of "food desensitization" treatment that will help your body learn to tolerate the specific foods troubling you. In my experience, desensitization is unreliable and unrewarding at best. Any food to which you have been found to be reactive can be "tamed" to a very limited degree if at all, and repeated exposures to it through desensitization might perhaps make your arthritis reaction greater rather than smaller. I am also highly skeptical about the value of skin testing and patch testing as means of identifying the causes of your allergic reaction. This is because the test results are reportedly less than 50 percent accurate, with false positive and false negative findings turning up about equally. There is also the RAST (radioallergosorbent test of blood chemistry) and sublingual provocative tests (extracts of food placed under the tongue) for detecting food-related allergies. All these measures are costly and are still nowhere nearly as accurate for arthritis as testing foods by the FED.

I must say, however immodestly, that no alternative system I know of is intrinsically more reliable, less costly, or closer to the site of the allergic problem than the combination of the Food Elimination Diet and the Daily Pain Score. Together, they really give you a window on the problem as it is occurring, and an objective way of knowing when your immune system is functioning on your behalf and when it is causing unsatisfactory reactions.

The failure of food desensitization by shots brings another patient to mind. Jennifer W #7 was a 54-year-old woman who had endured 20 difficult years with severe fibromyalgia and who was receiving many shots for multiple food and environmental allergies. I placed Jenny on the FED, at the same time totally stopping the desensitizing shots. Her baseline total pain score of 54 promptly tumbled down a gratifying 78 percent, bottoming at 12. Her reactive foods were found to be wheat, sugar, milk, corn, eggs and tomatoes. Daily menopausal hormones were then used to transport her to a pain score of zero, a condition that understandably seemed to her like Seventh Heaven. All but 22 percent of her presenting illness was relieved by correct management of her food allergies; the remainder was relieved by controlling her hormonal immunity.

Here are some case histories which should fire up your enthusiasm for giving the Food Elimination Diet a try.

The first example is an 81-year-old patient I will call Maude O #8. When I first saw Maude, she had lived with rheumatoid arthritis for 20 difficult years. Conventional care by her rheumatologist had brought her no relief, and she was scarcely able to function. After a week of charting her Daily Pain Score, we pegged her baseline total pain score at an almost unbearable 162. I put her on prednisone immediately, and this brought the score down to 24. Maude thought, "Great job!" and might have been satisfied to leave well enough alone, but I persuaded her to start the FED. Her score promptly fell to zero and, except for brief flare-ups as she tested foods in Classes II to V, she has held to zero ever since. Her reactive foods were found, by the process of elimination, to be wheat, cheese, butter, coffee and pork. The coffee reaction will sometimes go away quickly rather than slowly. She no longer needs prednisone.

My next example is Patricia O #9, who was both considerably younger (age 37) and in much less pain (score 21) when she began my treatment, but the relative degree of improvement she underwent as a result of the FED was identical. As the result of eliminating coffee, wheat and dairy products, Patricia's rheumatoid arthritis pain score is now zero, week in and week out.

Good as the FED is, it does not detect all allergens. Some allergens are environmental, some are a bit of both. I am reminded of the odd case of Bill S #10, a 31-year-old tradesman who came to see me about his rheumatoid arthritis. Bill reported that in the course of about six months he had developed painful swelling of his hands, feet, ankles, shoulders and back. He was miserable. We pegged his baseline pain score at 46. I talked with him about the ways in which I thought he should go about isolating the cause of his arthritis, starting with the FED. Bill indicated that he found the idea of dieting almost as bad as the pains, but he did agree to stop chewing his plug of tobacco, a pleasure he had taken up about nine months earlier. Within one week of stopping the tobacco, Bill's pain score dropped to zero. The only time he had a glimmer of pain was when he smoked a cigarette or went into a smoke-filled room, and then his pain score would go up five or tens points by the next morning. It didn't take a genius to recognize that for Bill, tobacco was the "food" causing his problems. And second-hand smoke, which Bill ingested though his nose and mouth, turned out to be nearly as toxic as any conventional food that might trigger arthritis.

Molds, chemical pollutants, auto emissions, insecticides and chemicals found in building construction materials are other sources of environmental allergens that the FED is not capable of detecting, but which, regrettably, may be a causative factor in some people's inflammatory reaction. If, after you have carefully explored the FED approach, you suspect that some other environmental agent could be involved, you had best see a bioecologist physician, who will investigate these areas.

Edith C #11 was 63 years old when she first hobbled into my office. She had been a schoolteacher, and was forced to retire very early by her rheumatoid arthritis, which had started twelve years previously. Her central problem was severe bilateral knee involvement with pain, swelling and redness. Gold shots helped a little for a few years, but then had to be discontinued because of a skin reaction. Plaquenil did well for a while, but then started affecting her eyes. She used large quantities of aspirin. Prednisone in large doses had been started one year previously and then dropped to 5 mg daily. X-rays reportedly showed changes of both knees, so bilateral knee joint replacement was planned.

When Edith started her treatment with me, her baseline score was 23. A prednisone induction brought the score down to 12. When she did the FED, the score went down to 4. Eggs were found to be the major reactant food, but there was also some mild reactivity to yeast and cheese. The foods detected to be reactive were subsequently meticulously avoided, and over the next two months her numbers gradually went down to zero. Every bit of the redness and swelling went away. There are occasional small flares of pain that are quickly brought back to zero by Microdose prednisone. With no pain in her knees, Edith can now walk anywhere with agility, she has resumed her gardening, and she wishes that she were back in teaching.

Barry C #12 is a 75-year-old retiree who occasionally plays duplicate bridge with me. His psoriatic arthritis made it almost impossible for him to move from table to table and to hold his cards. He wore protective elastic material for his wrists and elbows. He heard that I was interested in arthritis and inquired what could I do. We first established his pain score to be 46. With the FED diet his score slipped down for three weeks to zero, and stays there. The offending agent was proven to be coffee. His psoriasis, which did not improve, was completely asymptomatic, so he opted to not take the B12 shots.

Amy B #13 was a 52-year-old office worker when she fist came to see me. Rheumatoid arthritis, present for 12 years, involved her hands and feet most prominently, but also her sholders, low back and knees. NSAIDs were of no value, but cortisone shots helped her feel better.

Amy's total pain score was 63 in 32 joints. The FED found her reactive to soy beans, bananas and white potatoes. By carefully adhering to the diet, Amy was able to keep her score mostly at zero, though she occasionally needed Microdose prednisone to cover slight flares of pain.

Now that you've seen how the Food Elimination Diet works, and the wonderful relief it can bring to so many, I hope you will agree with me that there is really no good reason not to give it a try. Even if you are being treated simultaneously for some other medical condition—cancer or diabetes, for example—you may be able to apply this diet to relieve your arthritis, so long as you do not violate the medical requirements of the other disease in doing so. It is imperative to obtain the assistance of your diabetes doctor if you are taking either diabetes pills or insulin injections, because you might have to make adjustments to the somewhat altered diet.

It would be of value for people with arthritis to repeat the FED evaluation at least every ten years to verify that no new reactant foods have developed in the intervening time.

REMEMBER

1. At least 25 percent of all arthritis patients are reactive to certain foods because their immune system has mistakenly, unpredictably and unalterably identified the substances as alien.
2. The Total Pain Score is the most reliable index by which to measure your reactivity to food and other reactive factors.
3. To establish whether you are part of that food-reactive group, you must take a test diet with a very low potential for reactivity for seven days. If you find that your total pain score drops, you assume with assurance that a reactive but as yet unidentified food has been removed.
4. Reactivity to a specific food is determined by an elevation of

your pain score coincident with eating that food for two days; nonreactivity, by no pain score change.

5. Your final, customized Food Elimination Diet (FED) consists of a diet that has eliminated only those foods to which you have demonstrated reactivity. All other foods may be eaten as part of your normal dietary pattern.

6. The pain relief achieved as a result of the FED may vary from zero to 100 percent.

7. Partial symptom relief by the FED suggests that some other immune factor may also be contributing to your residual pain.

8. Food allergy and hormonal allergy can produce the same pattern of arthritis pains, either separately or in combination.

9. I consider food desensitization regimens to be of no or even negative value in arthritis.

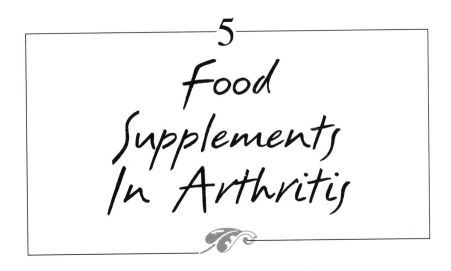

5
Food
Supplements
In Arthritis

SPECIAL HELPMATES TO MEET SPECIAL DEMANDS

I MENTIONED earlier that no food that you can eat will prevent the appearance of arthritis, and no food can cause its onset unless you are individually allergic to it. Likewise, your weight is not a critical factor in the onset of rheumatic inflammation, with the exception of gout, in which obesity does seem to be a provocative factor. (Excess weight can, however, put extra mechanical strain on joints that are already in trouble.) It is also true that all your ordinary basic nutritional needs are met by a normal, healthy diet. However, food supplements can be valuable in meeting the special demands of your arthritis condition. Also, as we progress past the age of 40, various protective systems of our bodies wear down a bit and need additional help. While there are numerous supplements to mention, I shall describe only those items that are readily available commercially and are of reasonable effectiveness, safety and cost.

VITAMIN B12

Vitamin B12 (cyanocobalamin) is a water-soluble vitamin found in small amounts in legumes (beans, peas), but mostly in meats, particularly pork. B12 must unite with a substance made by your stomach called the intrinsic factor in order to be absorbed into the wall of the intestine. The B12 is then transferred to another carrier, called transcobalamin-II, and stored in the liver until needed elsewhere. The large stores of B12 in the liver will keep the body functioning normally for several years after additional dietary supplies have ceased. Even if your liver loses half of its B12 , it is still able to maintain a normal level of the vitamin in your blood for an extended period. The B12 functions as a metabolic enzyme, critical in the reproduction of DNA and cell growth. Vitamin B12 depletion leads to the red blood cell disease called pernicious anemia, and its deficiency also leads to such nerve tissue problems as numbness and paralysis (Harrigan and Heinle 1952).

We have the ability to measure the blood levels of B12 in the laboratory, and a person found to have normal levels is generally considered healthy in this regard. However, I have found that these ''normal'' blood levels are not always reliable in patients who are functionally deficient in B12. The particularly troubled patients develop localized requirements for higher levels of B12 in one or more groups of tissues. I call this problem focal B12 hypovitaminosis, or focal elevation of a specific tissue threshold. In order for that one particular tissue to function effectively, your entire body must have a higher-than-normal level of B12. The following case report should give you a clearer understanding of my B12 concept.

My friend Gary C #14 was 70 years old when he was admitted to the hospital under the care of other doctors. Gary, a businessman, had a six-month history of indigestion, occasional vomiting, right upper quadrant abdominal pains and recurrent chills with fever. The laboratory revealed several types of bacteria growing in his blood, an extremely serious condition. X-rays demonstrated gallstones, and laboratory tests further revealed evidence of an inflamed pancreas. Gary was given appropriate antibiotics for one week, and then he underwent surgery for the removal of his gallbladder.

For the next 52 days, neither food, fluid nor X-ray dye passed through Gary's stomach into his intestine, though the opening into his intestine that should have made such passage possible appeared normal, and he had to be fed intravenously. His physicians tried every conceivable medicine to solve the stomach problem, but unsuccessfully. At the end of 52 days, Gary underwent another operation, this time hooking up his stomach through a new opening into his intestine to bypass the supposed obstruction. Once again, he experienced no improvement at all in the passage of anything through his stomach. Now he was growing so weak that he required five blood transfusions to stay alive. Throughout this time the culture of his blood, urine, bile and incision were checked regularly; they indicated the presence of the three kinds of bacteria, none of which seemed to be diminished by antibiotics. Gary's condition continued to worsen until his kidneys and liver were found to be failing. Death seemed certain, and he was administered the Last Rites.

All the while, Gary's B12 determinations were normal and he received 1 microgram B12 daily in his central alimentation. I suggested to Gary that he ask his doctor to give him 1,000 mcg of B12 by injection, a thousand times the recognized daily requirement. Gary's doctor was predictably angry and resistant to this suggestion; but, with Gary's pleading and a reminder that his outlook was otherwise exceedingly bleak, the doctor reluctantly agreed to fulfill a dying wish—Gary got his B12 shot.

Within 24 hours, Gary's temperature returned to normal and he was able to drink liquids for the first time in 77 days. Within 48 hours he started foods and within 72 hours he had his first spontaneous bowel movement. Signs of infection were no longer detectable either. After a few more days Gary left the hospital and returned to working full time in his business. About every three weeks his digestive system began to act up, a sign he took to mean that he needed another B12 injection, administered by his family, to keep healthy. He has sensibly followed that injunction ever since.

My explanation for the success of B12 therapy has two parts. First, the extra B12 Gary received restored the action of the autonomic nerves that run the muscles of his digestive tract so that the intestines could get back to their normal function. And second, the elevated levels of B12 invigorated the immune system, enhancing the ability of the lymphocytes to make antibodies and of the macrophages to eat and destroy the invading bacteria in coordination with the antibiotics.

Five years after recovering from his digestive disorder, Gary developed a new medical symptom—severe pains mostly in his lower back, but also in many joints. After expensive, extensive investigation, his physician diagnosed his pain as coming from spinal stenosis, a narrowing of the bony column enclosing the spinal cord. The problem was considered not appropriate for surgery; pain management was offered as the only alternative, but ordinary painkillers did not help much. His only hope, his doctor said, was to control the pain through narcotics. Before Gary would subject himself to such a drastic approach, he came to me for another opinion. Before making further recommendations, I asked Gary to take a week to establish his total pain score.

Gary reported that his daily pain score averaged 84, from many joints. On the basis of the widespread distribution, I was convinced that he was suffering from arthritis. Playing a hunch, I asked him to pay particular attention to what happened to his pain directly after his regular triweekly B12 injection. Gary reported that it gave him very good pain relief for about two days. I then recommended that he take the B12 shot every two days; when he did, his pain score dropped to a more tolerable 40, without any assist from narcotics. By my reasoning, Gary's original medical crisis had come as a result of the inability of his immune system to fight bacteria, and his new problem had developed because of his body's inability to destroy immune complexes, problems both addressable in his case by supplemental B12.

Why not take B12 by pill, you may ask? B12 must be taken by injection to overcome three potential problems. The first is the possibility that the body lacks sufficient intrinsic factor from the stomach to promote the large absorption of B12 into the blood at anything even approaching normal levels. Second, even if there is ample intrinsic factor, there will still be only enough to maintain liver supplies and a "normal" blood level; the need for local, special surpluses will not be met. Third, circulating blood supplies of B12 in excess of normal are excreted rapidly in the urine, so that even the excesses of 1,000 mcg by shot last only 24 to 36 hours. Consequently, the only way to provide abnormally high levels of B12 is to bypass the intestinal tract. When the bloodstream is flooded with the vitamin by injection, the cells of high-threshold tissues fill up to their maximum and are able to coast for two days to three weeks—until the need for more vitamin B12 surfaces again.

The injectable form of B12, which I teach my patients to give themselves at home in the same way diabetics do, is available only when prescribed by a physician. As mainstream medical groups discourage physicians from using B12 for anything other than treating pernicious anemia, you may find your doctor resistant to this approach. But don't accept defeat—look elsewhere until you do find a doctor with an open mind. I assure you that B12 is nontoxic and without negative consequences no matter how much you use. It costs 20 cents a shot to give it to yourself, but up to $30 when given by your doctor.

Another case report demonstrates the value of high-dose B12 in treating a number of health conditions. My patient Vanzy K #15 was 79 years old when she first came to see me for rheumatoid arthritis which, she said, had troubled her since the age of ten. She had tried gold and various NSAIDs at her doctors' urgings; but, except for aspirin, she received no relief. At age 59 Vanzy had both knees surgically replaced. At 77 a case of shingles left her with the constant, severe, burning face pain of post-herpes zoster neuritis, or nerve inflammation. Of all the therapies tried, including those of nationally prominent clinics, none had given her relief. She was also diagnosed with pernicious anemia, and for this she received monthly B12 1,000 mcg injections. There is an established, frequent association between pernicious anemia and rheumatoid arthritis (King 1992). When I asked her to specifically and carefully observe what happened after a B12 shot, she reported that for about three days afterwards she had no face pain at all.

Vanzy established her arthritis baseline total pain score as 38. Under a regimen of Microdose prednisone, her score went down to 15. At that point Vanzy started to self-administer B12 three times a week for complete control of her herpes pain. In about six to eight weeks she realized that coincidentally she no longer needed prednisone and that her total pain score was down to 6. Vanzy still needs her B12 shots regularly to keep her neuritis pain at bay. Ironically, I intentionally used the B12 for Vanzy's herpes pain, and serendipitously discovered its value in controlling her arthritis pain as well.

In time, I came to understand how to use high-dose B12 in healing arthritis. I now prescribe it for many of my patients in the following manner: I start each patient with a thrice-weekly regimen of B12 injections for three weeks. Let's say for purposes of demonstration that the pain score starts at 50. If the pain score is still 50 at the end of the three weeks, it is clear that B12 is not relevant in this case and we discontinue its use. If, on the other hand, there is a drop in the total pain score, we continue the B12 at the same frequency until the score drops no further and remains the same for at least one week, say at 20. Now we gradually increase the time between shots one additional day at a time until the pain score begins to rise again, for example to 23. We then know that the frequency used just before the score rise occurred is best for your individual case, be it every two days or every 21 days. Should subsequent changes occur, because of other factors such as stress or age, you can reassess your schedule to fit your needs. This system not only assures that you get the best results from B12, but also that you take no more than necessary for optimal control.

CHANGING B12 THRESHOLDS

The threshold changes for B12 seem to occur in only certain groups of tissues, not the whole body. I believe that I can identify two tissues that may be so affected, but time may prove that there are more:

The first tissue system identified as having an elevated B12 threshold is the immune system. When a group of experimental animals that were B12 deficient were injected with an exact dose of bacteria, they almost all died of the infection. When another group of the same animals that was well supplied with B12 was injected with the identical dose of bacteria, they almost all survived the infection. It has been demonstrated that when white blood cells that specialize in fighting infection are deficient in B12, they are subsequently less effective in engulfing and destroying bacteria. This probably explains the circumstances surrounding Gary C, who nearly succumbed to a total body infection, but recovered rapidly when much more than normal amounts of B12 were administered to meet his elevated threshold. Gary C's case was different from that of the deficient animals in that his blood levels were normal throughout his prolonged illness and he had been getting B12 1 mcg daily for weeks in addition.

The natural close relationship between B12 and phagocyte activity is suggested by the fact that phagocytes are the only cell group (other than the specialized intestinal cells that first absorb B12 in the body) that make transcobalamin-II for B12 transport.

It is well known that phagocytes consume and destroy bacteria, but it is less appreciated that they also consume immune complexes. I therefore consider that B12 gives major support to the primary inflammation defense system. (See Figure 2-1, page 21.)

The second tissue or system with occasional elevation of the B12 elevated threshold is nerve tissue. Nerves must have an adequate supply of B12 for function; without such, nerves will occasionally degenerate as they sometimes do in untreated pernicious anemia. Localized groups of nerves may be involved, as in Gary's intestinal malfunction. My high-dose B12 therapy evolved from recognizing that the successful experience I had in treating many older women for urinary incontinence due to bladder nerve malfunction might have parallels here in Gary. So too, my treatment of Vanzy K was an outgrowth of previous positive B12 experience in treating other sorts of pain, numbness, weakness, spasm and paralysis due to altered nerve function; I knew that the pain or numbness of hands and thighs in some of my pregnant patients had been nicely relieved in at least 90 percent of cases by B12 injections.

The combined development of arthritis and nerve damage shows up again in the case of Glenn B #16, a brilliant, 82-year-old retired diplomat when I first met him. Glenn told me he had endured osteoarthritis for 30 years, and that during the past 12 years, his most disturbing problem had been damage to many nerves of his hands and legs. He told me that the nerve trouble had produced a gradual progression from pain and weakness to numbness and paralysis. In spite of countless medical and neurological consultations, courses of physical therapy, and leg braces and splints, he was on a downhill slide. I noted immediately that when Glenn walked, he staggered, even though aided by a cane, because, as he later explained, he could not feel where his legs were. He could not dress himself, either, because he could not move his thumbs against his painful, stiff fingers. My examination confirmed numbness in his hands and a stocking-like anesthesia from four inches above his knees down to his toes. The reflexes of his knees and ankles were absent. We determined that his baseline total pain score from the arthritis was 52.

I immediately started Glenn on vitamin B12 1,000 mcg by injection daily and also vitamin E 800 International Units daily by mouth. In just 24 hours he experienced enough of an improved sense of touch in his hands so that he could button his own shirt. After 48 hours, he could move his muscles more easily, notably his legs, since he was starting to get neurological clues to where they were located. After 72 hours, his numb legs were starting to have some normal feeling again, his sense of balance improved and absent reflexes started to return. He could even think better, the result of better nerve connections in his brain. His total pain score dropped down to 36, and he felt fit enough to give a visiting lecture at a nearby university. After 96 hours, Glenn reported better sleeping and improving mobility in his right ankle, the first such voluntary motion in many years. After two weeks we were able to decrease the frequency of B12 injections to every two days.

Five weeks into therapy, Glenn's total pain score was down to 18. I then added oral vitamin B1 100 mg daily to further enhance phagocytosis and nerve function, and two weeks later his total pain score had sunk to 10. The once widespread zone of anesthesia was now localized in his feet only, and he was beginning to register a little pain there, a sign of sensation returning. But he was still unable to get good use of his leg muscles, which had been without voluntary motion for 12 years.

Glenn's paralysis and inflammation responded very satisfactorily to B12, and it is likely that they are representative of similar, focally elevated B12 thresholds, particularly in the absence of pernicious anemia. This brings up an interesting question: does B12 nourish the nerve directly to improve its function, or does the B12 enhance the body's defenses enough so that they can remove the immune complexes that would otherwise irritate the nerves and lead to dysfunction? Is it perhaps a combination of both? We just don't know, but meanwhile we can say that it has a very favorable effect on a serious problem. In Appendix A I will describe the Cyclic Anesthesia and Paralysis Syndrome, wherein paralysis and anesthesia are completely controlled by removing immune complexes without B12 manipulations.

There is a third important mechanism for the control of inflammation through the action of B12. It also happens to involve nerve tissue, specifically in the brain's hypothalamus, which, amongst several critical roles, is responsible for the release of hormones, including the anti-inflammatory cortisol. As inadequate pulses of cortisol are a factor in arthritis, and as B12 appears to be essential in the normal operation of nerve tissue, it is reasonable to propose that high doses of B12 might play a role in stimulating a lagging or dysfunctional hypothalamus to resume normal production of cortisol releasing factor (CRF). With larger amounts of CRF leading to satisfactory pulses of cortisol, greater control of inflammation is a natural result. I consider that the hypothalamic-cortisol response to inflammation represents the secondary inflammation defense system. (See Figure 2-1, page 21.)

Appearing to confirm this hypothalamus theory is the fact that patients receiving high doses of B12 commonly experience improved spirits and increased energy (Dunn and Berridge 1990). In the past, these changes were believed to be nothing more than a psychosomatic response to having a physician do something therapeutic for the patient burdened with chronic aches and pains. But there are now independent scientific data supporting the notion that increased levels of CRF improve mood and energy. It takes high doses of B12 to reach the elevated threshold. The resultant CRF improvement surely energizes the patient so treated and leads him or her to feeling better emotionally as well as reducing rheumatic inflammation.

I cite the story of Peter R #17 as still further evidence for the excellence of B12. Peter was a 75-year-old retired optician when he first came to see me. His osteoarthritis of 30 years had resisted all standard rheumatological medications. He had recently been diagnosed as having had a mild stroke. He needed assistance in getting out of his wheelchair because of pain, weakness and limited muscular control. Walking just a few steps was very difficult. His speech was slow and slurred. Not surprisingly, he felt depressed and withdrawn much of the time.

Peter determined his baseline total pain score to be 25. I started him on the FED, but no improvement occurred. Curiously, when I tried a standard prednisone induction, his pain score rose to 30, and the use of methylprednisolone, a related corticosteroid drug, had the same adverse effect. Nor did spironolactone bring any relief.

When I decided to prescribe shots of vitamin B12 1,000 mcg three times a week, he began to experience a rapid improvement. Not only did Peter's muscular strength increase by 50 percent so that he could get out of the wheelchair by himself, but he could walk. Peter also felt better emotionally. When he phoned me to report his progress, he seemed a new person that I could not recognize other than by name, because of his strong voice, normal talking speed and clear enunciation. When Peter's pain score plateaued at 12, I advised him to gradually spread out the intervals between injections until he found the minimal frequency that would still maintain his improved health status.

All told, Peter's vitamin B12 therapy had produced successful outcomes in three critical areas: his pain score was reduced 52 percent (inflammation control), his muscular strength was increased 50 percent (control of peripheral nerve irritation), and his thinking, coordination and mood were 90 percent improved (control of central nervous system irritation). Behind these changes, undoubtedly, are enhanced disease-fighting capabilities in the immune system, enhanced nerve transmission in the nervous system, and enhanced activity in the hypothalamus with resulting increases in cortisol and an elevated mood.

In summary, I recommend high doses of vitamin B12 as a nontoxic agent for the treatment of rheumatic disease. It must be given as frequently as your unique pain response dictates. As I have stated earlier, arthritis arises at least in part as the result of cell tissues developing elevated thresholds for B12 for which the body's natural and normal supply is inadequate. High-dose B12 therapy, in meeting the elevated thresholds of nerve tissues and macrophages, enhances their normal metabolism and function. In my experience, patients have a 60 percent chance of responding favorably to B12, and those who do respond experience an average of 55 percent reduction of their total pain score.

I would like to conclude my thoughts on B12 by referring you to *Dr. Wright's Guide to Healing with Nutrition* by Jonathan Wright, M.D. Dr. Wright treats painful bone spurs, bursitis and sciatica with daily shots of B12 1,000 mcg. He also treats active herpes zoster similarly, but does not mention his experience, if any, with the post-herpes pain syndrome. Nor does he explain why the medication works, stating only that he finds it of great value empirically. I welcome his company in this world of medical doubters.

Other Dietary Additives or Supplements

Vitamins are complex chemicals essential for the normal functioning of the body. With a few notable exceptions, the body takes in its vitamins through various dietary sources, including food and food supplements. The role of vitamins once absorbed into the body is partly but not fully understood, but through the evidence of what happens to health and bodily functions when any one of them is deficient, we can piece together some of their actions on one or more body systems or functions.

Following a normal diet usually provides us with all of our vitamin requirements, making vitamin supplementation not only unnecessary but possibly counterproductive to good health. But there are times when either because of stress, such as in infection, pregnancy or surgery, or when some process such as rheumatic disease occurs, supplements can be essential to recovery. Let me run through the more important vitamins and discuss what they can do for you or someone you know with rheumatic disease.

VITAMIN E

I have been using vitamin E regularly and as a good friend for the past forty-five years. During most of those years, vitamin E was referred to disparagingly by my medical associates. Then about two years ago researchers at Harvard University Medical School published a report on the value of vitamin E in reducing the risk of myocardial infarction, or heart attack, by 50 percent. Vitamin E's benefits derive from its activity as an antioxidant. Antioxidants block the action of oxidants, negatively charged chemicals that cause oxidation and thereby set in motion chemical events that can damage cell membranes, producing a host of long-term consequences inimical to good health. Cell wall damage produces inflammatory and troublesome prostaglandins. The comparative protection afforded by vitamin E and the NSAID aspirin against oxidative damage in the oxidation-prostaglandin cycle is diagramed in Figure 5-1.

In heart attacks, vitamin E intercedes in a chain of events that causes the adverse buildup of fatty deposits in arterial walls and eventually to coronary vessel clotting. In arthritis, which is our chief concern here, vitamin E inhibits certain chemical processes that eventually lead to the formation of prostaglandins, a group of hormone-like substances that cause pain and the inflammation which damage tissues. Unlike aspirin and NSAIDs, which also stop the formation of prostaglandins and produce stomach ulcers and kidney damage when taken over long periods or to excess, vitamin E causes no known problems under any circumstances.

Vitamin E is stored in part in the cell walls where it lies in wait to neutralize oxidants. The storage supplies of E can be used up in

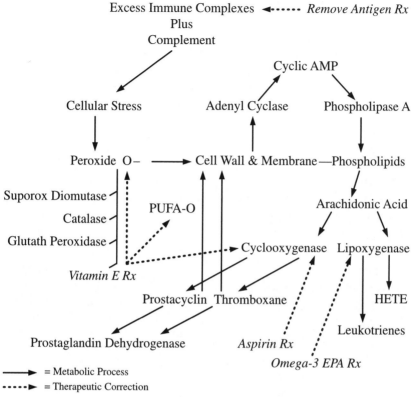

Figure 5-1. The Arthritis-Prostaglandin Cycle

performing this job, and, if they are not properly replaced, the membranes become subject to severe damage. Adding more E to the diet increases the storage of E in the cells until we get to the point of maximal storage from about 1,600 I.U. of E daily. Additional E does no more good, but it also does no harm.

I recommend at least 800 I.U. daily for arthritis patients. E is by far my favorite agent for the prevention of unusual clotting or inflammation which may occur in heart attacks, strokes, hemorrhoids and varicose veins. E tends to maintain normalcy, the middle of the road, which is the best place to be for neither unusual clotting nor unusual bleeding, and it thereby outshines aspirin. I also believe that vitamin E is superior to coumadin.

Vitamin E does much of its essential work in your joints, where it controls prostaglandins for reduction of inflammation. Another area in which E is effective is in the immune system where, like B12, it enhances the ability of phagocytic scavenger cells to gobble up and digest bacteria and immune complexes. The symptom change that you notice from taking E may be very modest indeed, but occasionally it is big. To my way of thinking, even if it does nothing apparent for your arthritis, the fact that it is so protective against unusual clotting, cataracts and arteriosclerosis, all of which are demonstrated benefits, makes it worthwhile. E also tends to control nighttime leg muscle spasms and to add extra walking miles to elderly or aching legs. Thanks to E, women enjoy diminished breast irritation and even some breast cancer protection, as well as decreased PMS discomforts. The goal of this simple type of therapy is not necessarily to conquer the rheumatic disease with a single agent, but to have each member of the body's therapeutic team do its part in achieving the best health and pain control possible. I often prescribe selenium, a trace element, as well, because it works synergistically with E as an antioxidant to keep blood vessels soft. The usual dosage of selenium is 100 to 200 mcg daily.

EICOSAPENTAENOIC ACID

Known commonly as EPA, or fish oil, this supplement is generally accepted in medical circles to be of benefit in the inflammatory process of arthritis. Although this product is sold as EPA, it actually consists of EPA and DHA (docosahexaenoic acid) which are helpful omega-3 fatty acids. EPA also affects prostaglandin metabolism, but in a little different way than vitamin E. (See Figure 5-1, page 69.) It diminishes the enzyme lipoxygenase so that there is a smaller production of irritating chemicals called leukotrienes. Similarly to E, EPA also diminishes the clotting of blood by interfering with the clumping of blood platelets, only it tends to do it more intensively. The resulting less-viscous blood flows more easily through narrowed vessels, which is especially good for heart and brain blood vessels narrowed by arteriosclerosis. Eskimos, who naturally consume large amounts of EPA in blubber, tend to bleed more easily when cut, but they also have fewer heart attacks. The usual recommendation is three to six capsules daily, but I find that one or two capsules daily conquers the problem of pain in my legs when walking. Again, the influence of this simple, mild agent on your total pain score is usually slight.

Vitamin C

Vitamin C, or ascorbic acid, maintains bones, cartilage, teeth and gums, helps to heal cuts and wounds, and promotes resistance to infection. It is also an antioxidant, helping to reduce the tissue damage associated with aging and to lower the risk of many cancers and heart disease. The regular use of vitamin C is very important for the prevention of scurvy, a deficiency rarely seen in industrialized nations, but still a concern for those eating inadequate amounts of fruit and vegetables. There are variable recommendations for the dose of vitamin C, but when a person is confronted with a chronic disease state such as arthritis, I think 1,000 mg daily is a good starting place, though there are those who take 5 to 10 grams a day. Some people develop diarrhea with C until they become adjusted to the large doses. I look upon C as an agent that helps reconstitute and conserve vitamin E after it has functioned in its antioxidant role. C enhances the function of the immune system and controversially prevents colds.

Beta-Carotene

Another good defensive weapon against oxidation is beta-carotene. Beta-carotene is converted into Vitamin A as needed. As long as the recommended daily supplement of 25,000 I.U. is not exceeded, there are no toxic effects to be expected, though this large dose should be avoided in pregnancy.

Vitamin B1

Vitamin B1, possibly better known as thiamine, is a water-soluble vitamin that functions in the metabolism of glucose for the production of

energy. Without this energy, bodily systems lose their ability to carry
out their many critical functions, such as the ability of the immune
system to swiftly ingest and digest foreign substances. Severe deficiencies of B1 can lead to weakness, numbness, brain dysfunction, heart
failure and ultimately death. Beriberi, which is seen today in people
with a very restricted diet, including alcoholics, is attributable to thiamine deficiency. As an obstetrician, I have discovered thiamine deficiency to be the basic cause of toxemia of pregnancy.

My evidence for an elevated thiamine threshold is not as strong
as that for B12; but, in the case of Glenn B #15, discussed earlier,
there was at first a substantial drop in the pain score from 52 to 20
with the use of B12; and then, after thiamine was added, the pain
score dropped further to 10. Whatever the mechanism may be, thiamine in much greater doses than normal seems to have enhanced
control of Glenn's inflammatory process. In addition to pain improvement, Glenn had a further surge of nerve improvement after the
thiamine was separately introduced.

The recommended daily allowance of thiamine is 1 mg. In a
well-fortified prenatal tablet it rises to 1.7 mg. The thiamine tablets
I recommend are 100 mg! Your supply of them will cost less than
three cents apiece, and it is virtually impossible for you to take too
much thiamine.

GLUCOSAMINE SULFATE

Glucosamine sulfate, as an aminomonosaccharide, is one of the basic
chemical constituents of the disaccharide units of glycosaminoglycans
and proteoglycans which make up joint cartilage. It is a small molecule that is easily absorbed, easily distributed to the body and readily
used metabolically. The favorable anti-inflammatory action of glucosamine is not by direct inhibition of the biosynthesis of prostaglandins
as with the NSAIDs, but it is reported to induce the synthesis of
glycosaminoglycans by cartilage cells, to protect the cartilage against
destructive enzymes, to reduce the generation of superoxide radicals
by macrophages, and to protect the cartilage against metabolic im-
pairment by the NSAIDs (Vidal y Plana et al. 1978). Proteoglycans
may stabilize cell membranes and intercellular collagen, thereby

being of antireactive ability or protective of cartilage. It makes little difference whether glucosamine is used in its hydrochloride or sulfate form. When incorporated into cartilage it is as glucosamine-6-phosphate.

Glucosamine is derived from the chitin in crab shells and from ground-up chicken cartilage. Shark fins reportedly supply chondroitin as well as glucosamine. The bones of sardines will not supply enough for therapeutic value.

The usual dose is 500 mg three times a day, and there have been no side effects other than transient intestinal discomforts. Your natural production of glucosamine is believed to diminish with age, and it is likely that larger amounts than normal are required to counteract the destructive influences of inflammation at any age. Therefore, oral supplementation is required at the times of symptomatic joint manifestations.

Glucosamine has been used for more than 30 years in osteoarthritis, and has relieved some of the pains, inflammation and stiffness, and replaced old, damaged cartilage with healthy cartilage. Clinical investigations reported in the medical literature vary greatly as to the degree of arthritis relief afforded by glucosamine. The ''miracle cure'' reports cited in Dr. Theodosakis's *The Arthritis Cure* suggest a 67 percent relief of pain overall, but the more sober observations I have found indicate that glucosamine is equal to or perhaps a little better than NSAIDs in pain relief, but about 100 percent safer from its lack of side effects. American pharmaceutical companies perform excellently controlled, short-term clinical NSAID evaluations and have claimed as much as 28 percent average pain relief. If glucosamine is equal or slightly better, its expected relief rate would be in the range of 28 to 32 percent. The relief it provides lasts for one to three months after medication is stopped.

Theodosakis also claims that chondroitin added to glucosamine will magnify the already miraculous results, but I am unable to find literature reports to substantiate that viewpoint.

An example of potentially misleading reports: An Italian investigator obtained 73 percent average pain relief with glucosamine—great! However, those who received a placebo were 41 percent improved! The actual benefit from glucosamine was only 32 percent—good, but not as great as it seemed at first.

I believe that glucosamine will be of ancillary value for clearing up some residual arthritis discomforts, but only after the basic removal and control of the antigens, as described in my book. It is far better to pull out the thorn in your foot than to take medicine perpetually to relieve the pain it produces!

MELATONIN

Melatonin is a hormone produced by the tiny pineal gland of your brain and by your intestines. It acts as a strong antioxidant and is a stimulator or rejuvenator of the immune system. Its natural production is usually markedly reduced by the age of 45, which is also the age at which the first indications of arthritis commonly appear. There are no established adverse effects, even from huge, prolonged doses. It helps many people sleep better. Take 1 to 5 mg at bedtime to coordinate with the natural circadian production at night. There is more information in Chapter 7.

VITAMIN B6

I have hesitated to recommend vitamin B6, pyridoxine, routinely for arthritis, because neurological damage can be done by excessive doses, say above 500 mg daily. Some authorities report that 200 to 400 mg daily will have a very favorable influence on carpal tunnel syndrome, an inflammatory condition associated with repetitive hand motion such as operating a computer keyboard; other good authorities doubt such claims. My view is that the recommended dose of 200-400 mg daily *may* remove the need for surgery for this condition without danger; and if it doesn't work, you have at least taken a protective measure against a possible excess of the amino acid homocysteine, a significant risk factor in atherosclerosis.

To give you an expanded sense of the power in controlling rheumatic disease that may lie in some of the simple dietary additives we have been discussing, let me cite the case of Margot G #18. I first saw Margot when she was 64 years old. Her rheumatoid arthritis had been present for the previous 12 years. NSAIDs had been of some help in reducing her pain, but they irritated her stomach too much. A cortisone shot in her left ankle gave some temporary relief. She had been taking Premarin as hormonal replacement therapy since her hysterectomy at age 50.

Margot determined that her baseline total pain score was 53. I started her on a prednisone induction along with vitamin E, vitamin C and EPA. The swelling of her joints disappeared as the pain score rapidly went down to zero. And on the infrequent occasions when pain flared up again, she was able to knock it back with Microdose prednisone. Margot gradually came to realize that the vitamins were the essential helper in her pain control, because the return of pain and stiffness was always associated with her forgetting to take her vitamins for a day or two.

CALCIUM

A degenerative process that often occurs in a joint involved with arthritis is the erosion, fragmentation and reduced structural integrity of the bone. Diminished bone strength leads to susceptibility to fracture. To make matters worse, a painful joint induces its owner to use it less and to put less weight upon it. Inasmuch as reasonable activity, particularly weight-bearing activity, is important to the maintenance of strong bone structure, bones are further weakened by the enforced inactivity. Additionally, rheumatic disease seems to have a marked predilection for females, and this creates high-risk circumstances during and after menopause when estrogen supplies are markedly reduced. The loss of natural calcium from weight-bearing bones, a condition known as osteoporosis or porous bones, is particularly rapid in the first three to five years of menopause. In sum, arthritis, inactivity and menopause all gang up to destroy the strength of bones and to lead to possible fracture under minor degrees of stress. Hip fractures in elderly women are, sadly, a major cause of death.

The dietary addition of calcium has a counterbalancing effect on osteoporosis, but just how much and when it is most effective are still open to lively debate. At a time not very long ago, expectant mothers in the U.S.A. were given prenatal supplements including calcium to make their babies strong and healthy. The fetuses grew well, but the mothers commonly experienced severe nighttime muscle cramps that would go away only when the pills were stopped. We now know that the phosphate portion of the dicalcium phosphate in the pills actually had a deleterious effect on the mothers in that it inhibited their ability to absorb calcium rather than adding to the supply; the cramps were thus an indicator of lack of calcium. Eventually, prenatal pills were reformulated to contain phosphorus-free calcium. Babies are now equally strong and beautiful, but their mothers rarely cramp.

Milk contains a lot of calcium, but it also contains a large amount of phosphorus. Expectant mothers who drink large amounts of milk can get the same severe muscle cramps due to calcium shortage that the prenatal supplements once caused. Milk is an essential food for babies who can use that calcium, because their calcium/ phosphorus metabolism is different from grown-ups'. Milk can be part of a well-balanced diet for adults when consumed in small quantities, but I believe that it is not the ideal source of usable calcium for rheumatic people who want to protect their bones. Rather than milk, I suggest that you take a phosphorus-free calcium supplement such as calcium carbonate, gluconate or lactate to protect your bones. And to enhance its absorption, take the calcium supplement with a small amount of vitamin D, as in the over-the-counter product called Os-Cal Plus D. The suggested amount of calcium to take ranges on up to 1,500 mg daily and more. The bone-strengthening effect of your calcium supplementation is very small, but it is real. At the same time I suggest that you reduce your milk intake to an amount that accords with your personal likes, and not to some idea of nutritional necessity. If you are one of the many adults who are allergic or reactive to milk, you might consider as a good substitute the product called Vegelicious, available from your health food store. The manufacturers of Vegelicious claim their product is superior to milk in supplying your calcium needs because of its reduced phosphorus content.

The kingpin of bone calcium control in the menopausal woman, of course, is estrogen replacement, and this is ideally done as soon as the onset of menopause is suspected. Estrogen is the cement that holds the grains of sand together to make a stone wall. Without such hormonal replacement, the major portion of your calcium is lost in the first three to five years of menopause. Indications of the menopause may be found in hot flashes, unusual emotional irritability or depression, as well as irregular periods beginning sometimes as early as in the forties. Even with estrogen supplementation and other measures, some degree of gradual bone loss is inevitable, but with proper care you can slow it down significantly.

Even if a woman is already five years or more into the menopause and the major portion of her calcium has already been lost, I still recommend estrogen to preserve the calcium that remains and possibly to increase bone strength, however slightly. Indisputable proof that this belated therapy works for bones is not yet available, but even if there were no bone value to be gained from the estrogens, their value for other body maintenance for prolonged life and better quality of life, measured by fewer heart attacks and better emotional status, merits its use.

A new, FDA-approved alternative to estrogen in terms of retaining and rebuilding calcium in bones is Merck's Fosamax, which is not a hormone and reportedly has no significant negative side effects. Its long-term effectiveness is still to be determined. Nasal and injectable preparations of the thyroid hormone calcitonin have proved helpful in the treatment of bone fractures, calcium balance control, and the deforming condition of bone known as Paget's disease. Calcitonin is, however, of questionable practical value for osteoporosis. In my opinion, nothing comes close to estrogen.

VITAMIN D

Technically, vitamin D is not a vitamin but a hormone, since it is processed naturally in the liver and kidneys from chemicals activated by sunlight. Vitamin D is a fat-soluble chemical which we obtain in supplementary form mostly from irradiated milk and also from fish oils such as cod liver oil. Provitamin D is stored in the skin where the proper exposure to sun radiation converts it to previtamin D, which in turn is processed by the liver and kidneys into active vitamin D, or calcitrol. Calcitrol is well known to be a potent stimulator of calcium and phosphorus absorption within the intestines. It promotes bone growth, but it can also dissolve bone if given in too large doses. Calcitrol receptors located on phagocytes attest to its being essential for the normal functioning of your immune system.

A marked lack of calcitrol leads to osteomalacia, which is decal-cification of the bones. In growing children the bone softening and deterioration is called rickets, which is marked by rheumatic-like pains, generalized aching and tiredness, tenderness around the joints, sensory nerve malfunction, weakness of muscles, emaciation and death from exhaustion. Vitamin D and sunshine will clear up these symptoms, which have much in common with arthritis.

Vitamin D and calcitrol also have a connection with psoriasis, a disorder in which patches of affected skin grow ten times faster than normal; psoriasis is commonly associated with a form of arthritis called psoriatic arthritis. The pinkish-red lesions of psoriasis are usu-ally covered with scaly skin which can produce sensations ranging from itchy to very sore. Supplements of vitamin D or calcitrol can slow abnormal skin growth and speed up the counterbalancing pro-cess of skin maturation and shedding. The application of calcitrol ointment is notably effective also in skin wound healing, which en-tails increased skin growth. I consider these observations to be an-other demonstration that among therapeutic choices, those that come closest to normalizing natural body processes in the middle of the road (as vitamin E) usually produce the best effects with the few-est negatives.

It is important in arthritis therapy to make sure that you are neither deficient in nor taking an excess of vitamin D. Except during the darkest winter months, the daily D requirements for adults can be met by exposing the skin to normal amounts of sunlight. A daily intake of 400 I.U., which can be found in one quart of irradiated milk, should meet the needs of anyone who has a deficiency. Shut-ins and people who work nights are the most common candidates for a deficiency. Excessive use starts at 1,000 I.U. a day.

Rheumatology texts include vitamin D in the general group of substances promoting bone integrity, but vitamin D is not generally considered to be an agent for control of the immune and inflamma-tory processes of arthritis. Though it is a minority view, I believe that a lack of vitamin D can result in arthritis through deficient function of the phagocytes. Vitamin D shortage may be an uncom-mon reason for arthritis in our modern, well-fed society, but it is still a possibility that should be checked out. Remember that in trying to get to the bottom of arthritis, which has so many causes, you cannot discount any possibility until you have experimented with it. And vitamin D, however unlikely its involvement, deserves looking at—at the very least in those instances when pain persists after all other avenues have been explored.

A radio person of yesteryear, calling himself "The Cod Father," seemed to be aware of the connection between fish oils, vitamin D and arthritis, because he recommended cod liver oil as a curative.

Remember

1. With disease or with elevated tissue thresholds of the immune and nervous systems, some food supplements come to play critical roles in restoring and maintaining normal cellular metabolism.
2. Megadose B12, delivered by injection, may enhance the function of both the immune system and the general nervous system. Oral therapy is ineffective in this regard.
3. Vitamin E protects cell walls and membranes from oxidative damage, improves blood flow especially through the heart and brain, and enhances natural pain control.
4. EPA works alongside E to improve blood flow and pain control.
5. Vitamin C and beta-carotene are very important antioxidants.
6. Vitamin B1 is essential for nerve and phagocytic function.
7. Glucosamine may assist in healing of cartilage and provide some relief of inflammation by an unestablished mechanism which is believed different from antiprostaglandins (NSAIDs).
8. Melatonin is a nontoxic hormone, a strong antioxidant and an enhancer of immune system function, all good for arthritis control.
9. Calcium helps maintain bone strength, though estrogen is the prime controller of bone calcium in the menopause.
10. Vitamin D enhances bone calcification and macrophage function. It is a hormone essential for the normal activity of your immune system, which at times is a key factor for improving arthritis.

6
The Gynecological Connection

WOMEN'S UNIQUE VULNERABILITY TO SOME FORMS OF
ARTHRITIS

It is an established fact that most forms of rheumatic disease occcur two to six times more frequently in women than in men. I have investigated and come to the conclusion that the causative difference is related to the monthly ovulatory and menstrual cycles of the normal woman. Specifically, I have been able to target the ovulation-associated hormone progesterone as the frequent culprit. Even more to the point, I have connected progesterone to rheumatic disease through a specific autoimmune sensitivity rather than through its natural metabolic function.

Ironically, I have been able to do this not because of any expertise in rheumatology—I am a gynecologist, after all, with little training in the specifics of rheumatology—but in spite of my initial ignorance of the specialty's fine details. To begin with, my principle diagnostic measure was my patients' reports of their pain experienced in muscles and joints. Once in a while I had the supposed benefit of a rheumatologist's detailed diagnosis in my patient's folder, but in truth I found little use to such "aids." I treated all the variously named rheumatic conditions from the same starting point, and was generally rewarded with favorable responses. By the time I had become knowledgeable enough to recognize distinct forms of arthritis on my own, it was already apparent to me that the high-tech process of differentiation practiced by most rheumatologists was really overblown, if not actually detrimental to treating the patient effectively. It is one more example of the fact that it sometimes takes an outsider to come up with a fresh and truly innovative solution.

The one difference between me and most medical outsiders, however, is in being an arthritis sufferer myself; it has sensitized me to some of the symptoms and pain patterns of others. Many patients who are afflicted with a particular disease go to the library to study up on their illness, and I was no different. I wanted to be able, at the very least, to ask the right questions when seeking a specialist's help; so I too went to the library to teach myself about rheumatology as well as the associated areas of immunology, allergy, endocrinology, pharmacology and anatomy as they pertained to my condition. My studies were made somewhat easier by the fact that, as a professional, I had previously been studying the relationship between gynecology and autoimmunity, and already had a working theory of autoimmunity as a prime cause of premenstrual tension and other cyclic gynecological symptoms and pathology. The fact that arthritis symptoms often responded to therapy using synthetic progesterone (progestin) in the same way that gynecological symptoms did, ended up as more of an affirmation of my preexisting theories than as a surprise.

The first clue that there might be a connection between arthritis and female sex hormones came when I observed how often my patients' arthritis symptoms lessened or disappeared coincident with the startup of hormone replacement therapy at menopause. It was only a short time before I determined to try a focused attack against arthritis with these same drugs. When the strategy proved sound, I started measuring the parameters of treatment. I came to realize that there was considerable variation from patient to patient. For example, my patients varied in the number of days of progestin therapy they needed—from as low as 5 to as many as 25 per month—to maintain consistent control of symptoms. I also came to realize that some patients responded well to one drug manufacturer's progestin formulation but not to another. This confirmed another idea, that the therapy was related to the immune response rather than to a physiological or normal function response. Likewise, the fact that in some rare instances the patient actually experienced an increase in arthritis pain rather than a decrease with progestin indicated that the progestins were actively involved in the mechanism of disease production rather than simply acting in some anti-inflammatory manner.

Another pleasing and attractive feature I found in my progestin therapy, as contrasted with conventional approaches, was that once a menopausal patient was matched favorably with a particular progestin, she could continue to use it indefinitely without experiencing any decrease in relief of those symptoms. This continues to be true even among patients who have been following my regimen for more than 15 years.

By contrast, when I used the same system of cyclic hormonal medication to control painful periods in premenopausal women, some patients occasionally experienced a gradual loss of progestin effectiveness over time. I attribute this undesired occurrence to the development of a cross-allergy. I do not know why there is this difference in behavior between the immune systems of menopausal and menstruating women. This cross-allergy event concerns the fickle reactivity of the immune system to the shapes of progestins. Through my changing the progestin formulation, however, relief from dysmenorrhea usually returned until a cross-allergy would again develop several years later.

Fortunately, the six or more replacement progestins available to choose from nowadays make it possible to extend the time during which we can treat cross-allergy-prone premenopausal women almost indefinitely. It also means that for those women who have no such crossover problems, we can be far more selective in finding the formulation best suited to individual body immunity.

Over the decade or more that I developed this approach to treating arthritis, the results got better and better. Accumulating data indicated that more than half of my patients were reporting better than 50 percent decreases in their arthritis-associated pain. Had I been more experienced in rheumatology, I would have recognized immediately that such results were indeed remarkable, but I assumed in my innocence that the rheumatological specialists were doing at least as well as if not better than I, an outsider, was.

Long ago, the dermatologists, rather than the gynecologists, figured out the answers to autoimmune progesterone dermatitis (Hart 1977, Shelly et al. 1964), which was unrecognizably associated with body pain and controlled by removal of the ovaries.

> Let me give you now a vivid example of how my then-experimental therapy worked wonders. When I first took Marion J #19's case, she was 61 years old and worked as a surgical scrub nurse. She had had a hysterectomy many years earlier, and for the past ten years had been on estrogen replacement therapy. The estrogen therapy maintained her in good health until, over the course of a few months, she developed red, painful and swollen finger joints. The skin around her knuckles cracked open, and little skin nodules began to discharge a thick, white matter. Under the circumstances, Marion felt she had no choice but to retire from nursing, but I persuaded her to hold on while we tried adding Provera 10 mg daily for 14 days each month to her estrogen. Within the first month her hands had nearly healed, and in two months they appeared normal and were entirely asymptomatic. Happily, she no longer felt under pressure to retire and continued in the work she loved. Ironically, her health was so good that after a year she decided to stop the Provera. The skin and joint problems returned, only to subside again when she restarted the medicine.

HORMONE QUALITY VERSUS QUANTITY

As a gynecologist, my initial medical focus was naturally on maintaining the *balance of hormones*—working with patients to get the elusive, correct balance of estrogen and progesterone that would make their bodies work optimally. I have since come to the belief that it is not the balance or quantity of these hormones that is of primary importance, but their *quality* or immunogenicity. The immune complexes from any immune-reactive hormones will produce symptoms unless the body's defense system is able to overcome them. The quantity of the reactive hormone is of secondary importance, I believe, in that a larger dose of reactive hormone will manifest itself in the increased intensity of the arthritic pains experienced and in the greater number of joints involved. Conversely, any *nonreactive* hormone will be asymptomatic, regardless of imbalance or quantity.

Just what are these troublemaking hormones? Natural progesterone is made monthly by the ovary when an egg is produced. A good ovulation will be accompanied by large amounts of progesterone, a poor ovulation will have lesser amounts, and a failed ovulation will make none. If there is sensitivity to the progesterone, the best ovulation will produce the most painful period, a poor ovulation will make only mild pains, while failed ovulation will cause none.

The quality or structure of the progesterone produced by an ovary may vary importantly at different times in the menstrual cycle. The chemical structure is controlled by the variable efficiency of certain enzymes. The body may be reactive to one form of progesterone and not to another. This explains why some women have pain only at the time of ovulation, some only premenstrually, and some only during menstruation, while others have variable combinations of all three. The unlucky women have three weeks bad and only one week good!

The process of arthritis-rheumatic disease runs a very close parallel to primary dysmenorrhea (the pain, cramping and other discomforts that often accompany the menstrual period). This relationship becomes most apparent when arthritis pains occur only cyclically and simultaneously with the painful periods. This parallel concept is strengthened by the cyclic, simultaneous appearance of arthritis, dysmenorrhea and paralysis in the same patient. (See V M #53 in Appendix A). Again, the form of arthritis experienced depends upon hereditary factors.

The exact manner in which artificial progesterone or progestin works in therapy for control of arthritis and other autoimmune diseases is debatable. I propose two mechanisms. The first is that, when progestin drugs are presented to the body in sufficient quantity, they can halt the production of native progesterone by decreasing the body's demand for it. This process is called feedback inhibition. The second conceivable mechanism is that the replacement progestin may have a greater ability or affinity than the native progesterone to combine with the potential antigenic protein to form a potentially antigenic complex. In such a situation, if the replacement progestin is not recognized as alien, then the progestin-protein complex will trigger no antigenic activity. This process, which I introduced in Chapter 2, is called competitive binding or competitive blocking.

Rheumatic Disease Therapy with Estrogen and Progestins

There are two objectives in female hormonal therapy that are directly related to rheumatic disease. The primary objective is to prevent the formation of antigen, the root cause of inflammation and pain in joints and muscles; the secondary objective is to maintain bone strength and integrity. Remember that rheumatic disease is caused by several factors, only one of which is progesterone autoimmunity, so not everyone can be helped with their arthritis through hormone therapy. But just about every woman can benefit from good bone maintenance. Progestin therapy coincidentally decreases the incidence of cancer of the uterus and estrogen maintains the strength of the bones. A negative for the use of hormones is the occasional menstrual-type bleeding that some menopausal women may experience. This nuisance bleeding is almost always benign, since the incidence of cancer is reduced, but it must be followed by careful evaluation. I personally never found a patient in whom it was malignant. The cyclic bleeding tends to diminish and disappear with time.

A yearly physical examination, including breast examination and Pap smear, is an essential part of responsible self-care, and an occasional endometrial biopsy may be indicated if irregular bleeding persists. Another mild problem that may accompany hormone therapy is preperiod bloating and blues, but this may often be overcome by changing the progestin formulation.

The presence of cancer in any of the female organs, including the breasts, is considered by many authorities to be a contraindication for the use of female hormones. This is because the hormones could theoretically stimulate the growth of residual cancer cells lying dormant following cancer therapies. But it is also true that for some women hormone deficiency can seriously diminish the quality of life—hot flashes, arthritis, emotional depression, reduced brain function, marked drying and narrowing of the vagina, osteoporosis, bone fractures, urinary infections, urinary incontinence and increased heart and brain thrombosis. Throughout the years I have educated my cancer patients, in whom no detectable tumor remains, regarding the risks and benefits of progestin and have given them the choice. Among those who selected hormone supplementation, no one has regretted the decision. One patient opted to take the hormone supplement route following surgery for ovarian cancer. Seven years after making a full recovery, this patient was advised by a university medical team to *stop* the hormones! Returning to me for further consultation, I found that she showed no signs of adverse effects—only good effects. I recommended that she continue the replacement therapy. She is still very well fifteen years later.

Hormone replacement is also discouraged for women with a history of thrombosis (heart attack or stroke), thrombophlebitis or blood clots to the lungs. But here again I disagree. Regarding thrombophlebitis, there is hardly a woman alive who has never had a bout with hemorrhoids, the anal form of phlebitis. And concerning coronary and cerebral thrombosis, consider the article in *The Journal of the American Medical Association* (Bush et al. 1983), in which it was reported that women taking menopausal replacement hormones lived longer and better than those not taking them, for reasons that included reduction of heart attacks and strokes! Although my viewpoint is strongly in favor of using the hormones, this is an issue on which you have to weigh the evidence and make up your own mind. According to Kilmer S. McCully, M.D., estrogens reduce the amounts of homocysteine in the blood, which he believes is the most important precursor to arteriosclerosis, heart attacks and strokes.

I recommend that all my patients on hormones take them along with vitamin E 400-800 units daily and sometimes with fish oil (EPA) as well. These nutritional supplements diminish the risk of clotting and thereby further reduce the already low potential for heart attacks and strokes. But if you are still dubious about using hormones, perhaps the story of another of my patients, Irene G #20 might sway you.

When I met Irene, she was in her seventy-sixth year. She was reportedly suffering from a 40-year case of osteoarthritis and fibromyalgia. She also seemed to have something severely compromising her mental processes. When I greeted her with "Hi, how are you?" it took her about three minutes before she could think and answer "All right." When I said "You must have arthritis," it took her equally as long to answer "Yes." She had been to some famous clinics, but with no mental improvement; Alzheimer's disease was suspected.

Because of Irene's inability to communicate clearly, I could not determine her pain scores. I prescribed an estrogen replacement hormone 0.625 mg for days 1-24 of the month and a progestin hormone 0.35 mg for days 10-24. The changes which began to appear within a relatively few days were simply astonishing. Irene began to talk and think more normally. Her mood and engagement in life were markedly better.

After one month when she returned to see me, she was not only conversing clearly and rapidly, but by her own estimates her arthritis pains had lessened by about 40 percent. Able at this time to do a pain score with Irene, we found she was still high at 110, which would suggest that her original baseline had been in the intolerable vicinity of 185. But in addition to the continuing but reduced pain, Irene now reported some difficulty breathing, particularly when lying down, which suggested heart failure. My check of her lungs found them clear, but her ankles were somewhat swollen. I immediately put her on spironolactone 75 mg daily, a potassium-sparing diuretic, as a replacement for the water pill she was taking. This revised therapy turned the trick. Irene's difficulty breathing disappeared and her pain score diminished to a more bearable 58. When I added vitamin B12 1,000 mcg by injection, it fell further to 31 in only two days.

Irene G demonstrates in an extreme fashion how replacement hormones in the menopause can not only decrease rheumatic pains but have other quality-of-life benefits as well. Irene's experience also shows that, contrary to medical opinion, the pains of fibromyalgia, one of the more intractable forms of arthritis, can and do respond to therapy.

HOW TO USE ESTROGEN AND PROGESTINS

I generally start patients on only one new medicine at a time so that I can verify that it is being tolerated well, and I can also observe its specific good and bad effects. This rule usually applies to estrogen and progestin, which I also introduce separately. Through this practice, I found that estrogen alone can relieve arthritis symptoms in about 4 percent of my women patients.

The accepted "bone-holding" dose of the most commonly used estrogen, Premarin, is 0.625 mg, and I start with that dose for women aged 50 to 60. For women over 60, I go with a smaller 0.3 mg dose, because older women are likely to experience breast tenderness with the higher dosage. Later, after their system has adjusted, I am sometimes able to increase the dosage, but I would rather settle for half the dose than to scare anyone away from hormone replacement therapy entirely on the basis of an unpleasant beginning experience with breast tenderness.

The menopausal daily dose of Premarin is given days 1 through 24 of the calendar month and then stopped until the first day of the next month. The week off medication allows for a possible menstrual flow, but most of the time there is none at all. If the estrogen agrees with you, I suggest that you plan to take it for the rest of your life. The estrogen will keep your body and brain functioning better even as it adds to your life expectancy.

Progestin therapy requires somewhat more individualized attention, first, as to the specific progestin that works best for you, and second, as to how many days it must be used each month to obtain the best effect. Currently there are four different plain synthetic progestins readily available under the names Aygestin (norethindrone acetate), Micronor (norethindrone); Ovrettes (norgestrel) and Provera (medroxyprogesterone acetate). The oral contraceptives Demulen (ethynodiol diacetate), Ortho-cept (desogestrel), and Ortho-cyclen (norgestimate) contain three additional forms of progestin, but they are less adjustable for menopausal women since the pill is made as a combination with a dose of estrogen larger than we wish in the menopause.

The differences between the various progestins are produced by very slight bonding and structural changes in a relatively large basic steroid molecule. (See Figure 6-1.) Those slight changes can make a vital difference between how that molecule behaves metabolically and how it is identified by the ultraperceptive immune system. It boggles my mind that these lookalikes can act so differently, with

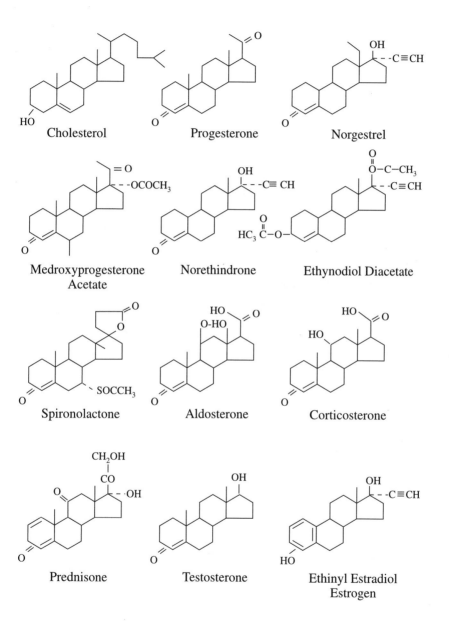

Figure 6-1. Steroid Chemical Structure

progesterone able to cause arthritis, norethindrone able to make it worse and norgestrel chasing all arthritis symptoms away!

Experience has demonstrated that patients may vary from 5 days to 24 days of progestin medication needed per month for maintenance of maximal symptom control throughout the month. One of my patients, Jessie W #34 (her case is discussed in detail in Chapter 8), goes so far as to take progestin virtually without cessation. She finds that if she goes more than two days without it, the painful symptoms return. Since she has had a hysterectomy and can use progestin without periodic breaks, she continues on. Normally, however, I start by prescribing 15 days of progestin medication for days 10 through 24 of the calendar month. If there is no change in the total pain score for one month, then a different progestin is used for the next month as we search for one that will be beneficial. If there is a drop in the total pain score, you then have evidence that the progestin is being helpful to your arthritis. You might want to try all the progestins, compare their benefits, and then select the one you like best.

If, on the other hand, the patient and I ultimately find no arthritis benefit, I still recommend that some form of progestin be continued indefinitely with the estrogen in the interest of general health, particularly for bone maintenance and protection from uterine cancer. When the progestin is being used purely for maintenance, however, I decrease it to days 18 through 24.

When you have selected the progestin that is most effective for you, you still need to do some further tweaking. Observe whether the pain score stays down throughout the month or whether it rises again before the time to restarting progestin medication in the next cycle. If the total pain score does rise, that indicates the need to start the progestin earlier, say days 7 through 24. If the pain score does not rise during the month, then try starting the progestin a day or two later. If your symptoms will allow it, bring the total number of medication days down to 7, days 18 through 24, for safe endometrium maintenance. Keep adjusting until you are satisfied the pain is managed most favorably for you.

The greater the number of days that you use a progestin in combination with estrogen in the calendar month, the greater your chance for irregular bleeding. With time and patience, and constant tinkering with the dosages, even heavy, irregular bleeding can often be solved. Such was my experience with Naomi G #21.

Naomi was a 54-year-old former nightclub performer. Her reason for coming to see me was related to her right knee. I could see that Naomi was in great discomfort, making it impossible for her to dance or even appear on stage. By way of explanation, she related that several years earlier she had been in an auto accident which had severely damaged her right knee. Following the necessary surgery, she had experienced constant pain, redness and swelling which neither standard medications nor physical therapy had been able to relieve. Reluctantly, she had to abandon her performing career to become a semi-invalid. I started Naomi on therapy with Premarin and Provera, and shortly after, she was ready to take a new lease on life. Not only were her joints and muscles moving more comfortably and easily, but she felt so good that she decided to go back to work on the stage. Because of her hormonal replacement therapy (HRT), she did begin to bleed rather heavily each month, but she was so grateful to her "little pills" that she would not even consider cutting back. She declared she would rather have a hysterectomy than give up the pills. Happily, such a measure soon proved unnecessary as her periods gradually diminished to little and then to none at all. Now, several years later, Naomi is still moving well, her arthritis under control and all but pain-free.

In rare instances, however, bleeding does become a problem to reckon with, when nothing that neither I nor time can do will stanch its flow. Patients then have the reasonable option of discontinuing HRT or having a hysterectomy. Most arthritis people would agree that a hysterectomy is far preferable to having the fierce and unrelenting pain return. Another method of bypassing the bleeding is to use the progestin alone, without the estrogen. This relieves the arthritis just about as well, but the multiple benefits of the estrogen are lost. As I tell my patients, whatever course of action you take in this regard is really a matter of personal choice rather than medical safety, one more compromise that must be worked out between what is and what you wish for.

The following case reports further demonstrate the powerful influence that hormones may have upon rheumatic pain.

Janice L #22, aged 50, came to see me because she was severely troubled by pains, tingling and numbness of her neck, shoulders and down her arms, especially at nighttime, when she had great difficulty sleeping. She failed to respond to the NSAIDs and cortisone of conventional therapy. X-rays showed bone degeneration, narrowed disc spaces and arthritic calcifications on both sides of her neck where the nerves exit the spinal cord. It seemed obvious to her managing physicians that the nerves were being pinched by the deformities and calcifications of her osteoarthritis. A neck collar and then a pulley traction at night provided minimal relief of pain and only limited sleep.

For Janice's problem I prescribed monthly Provera along with Premarin, and 100 percent of her symptoms promptly subsided. So did the need for traction, collar, physical therapy and pain medications. Repeat X-rays several years later showed the previous deformity and calcification pattern to be unchanged.

I believe that Janice's case is another instance of conventional medicine being on the wrong track both diagnostically and therapeutically. Regardless of the X-ray reports, it was obvious that there was no nerve pinching. It seems odd that both sides of her neck would be pinched at the same time. I believe that there was nerve irritation caused by immune complexes; and once the progesterone immune complexes were eliminated by the Provera, the symptoms simply went away. Likewise, the multiple neck calcifications were the result of immune inflammation rather than the cause of it.

My patient Dierdra L #23 was a 62-year-old widow who had had recurrent arthritis-type discomforts since the age of five, when she had recurrent fever and tender, swollen joints. All NSAIDs have had a limited, transient value and have produced prominent stomach distress. Prednisone 25 mg twice daily had produced no help for her asthma or her arthritis. She has received many allergy shots for dusts, molds and many foods. Histamine shots were of some value for her asthma. Her menopause occurred at age 54, and there had been a gradual worsening of the arthritis since then. Her diagnosis, established by a professor of rheumatology, was fibrositis. She had a low back spinal fusion in 1972.

Dierdra's baseline total pain score was 40; Premarin 0.625 mg days 1 through 24 and Provera 10 mg days 10 through 24 brought the total pain score down to 8 in one month and to 2 in the second month. The menstrual response to the hormones was a very heavy period accompanied by cramps, so the number of days of Provera was decreased to eight, days 17 through 24. Now the cramps and flow have been eliminated, and the pain scores average between 1 and 2. Dierdra also gave up her allergy shots and the foods for which she was theoretically being protected. Microdose prednisone is used for occasional small flares of pain which are produced mostly by vigorous muscular activity.

Fibrositis is well known to be unresponsive to standard treatment, and the therapeutic measure presently recommended for those patients is a fibromyalgia support group where the patients commiserate with one another. The great majority of my fibromyalgia patients have responded very well to various combinations of my therapies. Dierdra has had a lifetime of discomfort that was easily within the range of simple treatment, a combination of hormones, food and occasional prednisone.

Let me tell you about another patient with lupus who mystified all of her doctors by spontaneously getting completely better. Upon my review of her medical records, it became clear to me that her recovery was traceable directly to the commencement of her menopausal hormonal replacement therapy. Because Provera is not recognized in medical circles as being relevant to lupus, it was not even considered by her previous physician as being connected to her improved health. One is often blind to those things which are not being looked for. Unfortunately, hormonal therapy is not the magic bullet for all lupus, which can have a multiplicity of causative factors, either one at a time or in combination. But it is certainly worth a try in women who fit the profile.

REMEMBER

1. Immunity to native progesterone represents an autoimmune disease.
2. Hormone replacement therapy can relieve rheumatic disease that has a component of hormone reactivity.
3. The therapeutic effectiveness of a given synthetic progestin depends upon its immune nonreactivity quality rather than upon its quantity or hormonal balance.
4. Progestins work by halting the production of natural progesterone and/or by blocking its antigenic activity.

5. The number of days of progestin therapy necessary to constantly control rheumatic symptoms may vary from 5 to 25 days a month.
6. Estrogen in premenopausal women may be therapeutic by inhibiting ovulation; in menopausal women it also confers some protection to the structural integrity of bone. It enhances the longevity and the quality of life.

7
Other Hormones In Arthritis

THE MIGHTY MESSENGERS OF PAIN RELIEF

As a physician, I have always favored the natural approach over artificial and hi-tech modes when it comes to supporting and maintaining the health of my patients. To my mind, the most logical therapeutic agents to use in treating disease are those chemicals normally produced by the body in its own defense. Such agents include hormones, the body's chemical messengers.

Secreted in minute amounts by the endocrine glands, the hormones enter the bloodstream to travel to targeted areas around the body where they regulate and coordinate such critical activities as metabolism, growth and sexual reproduction. Over the past three-quarters of a century, we have also come to realize that deficiencies in these hormones can lead to a host of illnesses, including rheumatoid arthritis and dysmenorrhea.

Among the hormones of greatest interest to us are a diverse class of chemical compounds known as steroids, including the sex hormones progesterone, testosterone and estrogen produced by the sex organs; and the corticosteroid group, including cortisol, one of the nearly 60 chemical messengers produced by the adrenal glands.

Not until well after World War II was there any practical, inexpensive source of steroids for therapeutic use. Only the rich were able to get treatment, and not very good treatment at that. Equally important, because the chemicals were in such short supply, medical scientists were extremely limited by the small supplies of the product in the amount of research and clinical studies they could conduct in the therapeutic use of steroid hormones.

The situation began to improve when it was discovered that cholesterol, the fatty substance produced in the body and circulated in the blood, was a precursor of steroids. With some very complicated tinkering, biochemists found ways to alter the molecular structure of cholesterol to make various sex hormones, but scarcity and high cost remained factors prohibiting wide therapeutic use of the substances.

Then, in the 1950s, a number of scientific breakthroughs occurred that changed everything, including the outlook for patients suffering from rheumatoid arthritis. Heralded as a ''wonder drug,'' a cortisol-like chemical derived from animals and later plants was introduced. Called cortisone to differentiate it from cortisol, the natural corticosteroid of the adrenal cortex, the substitute was described at the time as ''the most complex compound ever marketed on a commercial scale.'' Cortisone's arrival was headlined in every major newspaper and medical journal in the country.

New as cortisone was, physicians were unsure as to how to use it either safely or effectively. Very large doses were used with initially very good results, but then adverse side effects started to become apparent. The developments ranged from cataracts, diabetes mellitus, exaggerated mood swings and stomach ulcers to facial swelling (the so-called moon face), humped back, osteoporosis, bone degeneration, hypertension, heart failure, generalized weakness, and arrested growth in some children. Because of these severe reactions, the initial promise of cortisone dimmed markedly over time. Used in proper doses and with discrimination, however, cortisone and its many corticosteroid variants are still wonder drugs.

Cortisol and synthetic cortisone work in the body to reduce inflammation in various locations by discouraging formation of prostaglandins, the natural fatty acids responsible for producing the pain and inflammation of damaged tissues. While reducing pain and in-

flammation is certainly a benefit, the price paid by large-dose cortisone users in terms of increased susceptibility to infection, the result
of impaired immune defenses, must not be minimized or forgotten.

Normally, your body produces cortisol on a rather reliable,
rhythmic 24-hour cycle, with the highest circulating blood levels occurring in the mornings between 8 and 9 A.M. and the lowest levels
occurring typically around midnight to 2 A.M. These levels, however,
are not sufficient to control inflammation, which requires a surge of
three to four times the blood level normally maintained. Such surges
of cortisol occur only under conditions of special stress, such as
surgical trauma, some major injury, or inflammation. At such a time
a messenger called Interleukin-1 (IL-1) goes to a tiny regulating
center in the brain known as the hypothalamus, and this becomes the
signal to produce an intermediary substance known as cortisol releasing factor (CRF). CRF sets in motion additional events that trigger
the production of cortisol, and with it the inflammation begins to
subside. If, however, the hypothalamus is stimulated too frequently,
as in the case of chronic arthritis, it becomes tired and unresponsive.
People with arthritis are reportedly very deficient in CRF production,
yet their circulating levels of cortisol remain essentially normal.

The cortisol replacement drug of choice for most inflammatory
symptoms today is prednisone. A hefty daily dosage of 5 mg of
prednisone at first tends to control inflammation quite well; but after
several months, many patients find they need 10 mg, and eventually
much more to maintain the same level of pain control. Unfortunately,
there is no amount of *daily* prednisone that will control the pain
permanently. And, with the continued high dose of corticosteroid
therapy daily, there is always the danger of one or more of the
adverse side effects mentioned earlier.

A BETTER WAY WITH MICRODOSE PREDNISONE

The new system of Microdose prednisone, upon which I have come
to rely, happily avoids virtually all of these toxic problems. It is
based on findings of Dr. Virgil Stenberg at the University of North
Dakota (Stenberg et al. 1992). Professor Stenberg demonstrated that

the response of body tissues to inflammation depends not on the mere presence of cortisol, which circulates in the blood at all times, but more particularly to a very large surge of cortisol which is several times higher than that in normal blood levels. Without the surge going above a certain threshold, Stenberg found, the inflammation remains unabated. He also determined that the sooner the inflammation is neutralized by a surge of cortisol, the less intense the inflammation becomes and the more rapidly it goes away. In other words, it is important to respond quickly to a new or increasing arthritis pain by "nipping it in the bud."

Basically, Microdose therapy, as I practice it, consists of a brief induction phase followed by a low-dose maintenance regimen. The standard induction phase, which involves relatively higher doses of prednisone, is designed to bring existing inflammation and pain under control, and is necessary whenever the baseline pain score is above 10. A prednisone dose of 5 mg or more inhibits hypothalamic function by feedback and allows it to rest. The induction phase usually lasts about three weeks.

The Microdose therapy that I use after the induction phase consists of five days on prednisone followed by at least five days off medication. The aim of Microdose prednisone therapy, then, is to mimic or replace the natural but intermittent CRF-induced surges, doing so as infrequently and with as little prednisone as will do the job. In this way the hypothalamus is given a chance to recuperate during 5-day dosage periods, its deficient CRF surges are replaced by prednisone, and then the rested hypothalamus is put back to work as the prednisone is withdrawn.

The Microdose prednisone effect works best when it is given at a time that coincides with the body's natural daily peak. Thus, if 5 mg prednisone is taken between 7 and 8 A.M., it is absorbed into the bloodstream just in time to piggyback on the natural circadian rise of cortisol that takes place in the mornings roughly between 8 and 9. The timing I use for prednisone is very different from the common directive to take prednisone in divided doses through the day, which makes it unlikely to produce a significant cortisol surge.

Based upon the experience of my patients, the five on-five off regimen allows the hypothalamus the three to five days it needs to recover. In many cases the routine works so well in reactivating the hypothalamus that pain scores actually decrease still further for a few days following withdrawal of medication. In these ways the Microdose system not only avoids the serious problems associated with continuous therapy, but it gives a greater, more dependable relief. And because the dosage is intermittent, it uses much less of the prednisone all told.

Among the many arthritis patients to demonstrate the validity of Microdose prednisone as a superior method, perhaps none makes a more dramatic case than Larry B #24. Larry was a 59-year-old farmer whose condition of rheumatoid arthritis started ten years ago. Many of Larry's joints were involved with pain, and X-rays showed damage to his hips and knees. He was also troubled by significant weakness, requiring him to use artificial supports for his right foot. NSAIDs were of some value in curbing associated pains; but, in the quantities he needed them, they produced acid stomach problems for which gastrointestinal drugs were of no countervailing effect. Larry was also on daily high-dose prednisone, which his physician had begun two years earlier at 20 mg daily and scaled back to 5 mg daily mainte-nance; the prednisone was giving only partial pain relief. Chills and fever also dogged him periodically. Understandably, Larry was miserable.

When Larry came to me, I gave him as his first assignment the filling-in of his Daily Pain Score chart. We found that his baseline score was 37. I then put Larry on the standard prednisone induction, and his scores went down to 4. This was followed by Microdose prednisone management to keep his score between zero and 6. I also urged him to stop drinking coffee. His use of prednisone averaged 1 mg per day.

Under the Microdose regimen, Larry not only got rid of his foot brace and muscle weakness but regained his old zest for life. He returned to farming, and during the winter season he moved to Colo-rado to ski! With the Microdose regimen, his daily prednisone intake was 1 mg, compared to the 7.5 mg of borderline safety. With 80 percent reduction in his prednisone intake he obtained more than 90 percent improvement in pain control. Six months after starting ther-apy, a tiny patch of psoriasis appeared and possibly changes his diagnosis to psoriatic arthritis.

The case of Marcia S #25 is equally encouraging. When I first saw Marcia, she was 56 and had been living with osteoarthritis for about nine years. She had been experimenting with various home remedies, but to no avail. When asked to rate her pain, she presented a total pain score of 36. Subsequently I put her on a prednisone induction, and her score promptly went down to zero. After she proved so responsive, she found the need to use Microdose prednisone only once every two or three months when a minor pain began to reassert itself. Each time, with the prednisone she quickly went back to zero.

In fact, Marcia felt so well that she thought she might be cured, leading her to do a little experimenting on her own. At the next sign of mild pain she took no medication. Over the ensuing month these pains gradually went back towards their starting point. When Marcia came back in distress, we did the induction all over again, and now she treats herself with Microdose cycles as soon as she experiences little pains, about every two or three months. My analysis of the mechanism at work here is that Marcia possessed a constantly depressed hypothalamus which, with the help of Microdose therapy, was restored to normal function for months at a time.

I also want you to meet Barbara J #26, who shows us that through the proper application of Microdose prednisone therapy the hypothalamus can sometimes recover some normal function even in an environment of constant pain, and even after previous huge doses had been to no apparent avail.

Barbara, a Native American, was 52 years old when she first came to see me. In taking her history, I learned that she had rheumatic fever as a child and that her rheumatoid arthritis had begun in her early forties. Since that time the disease had progressed in severity until every single one of her joints, other than her jaw, was in pain. Medically certified as totally and permanently disabled, Barbara was awaiting a place in a nursing home, because she could no longer take care of herself.

As Barbara's condition had worsened, physicians had tried all the standard therapies. NSAIDs were quickly discarded as of minimal value, one of which gave her hives on top of all her other troubles. Plaquenil, a drug used to treat severe rheumatoid arthritis and lupus, as well as gold shots, another favored but costly therapy, had also produced side effects that rendered them unacceptable. Over the previous two years Barbara had been given multiple cortisone shots in her knees, ankles and shoulders, but at best these gave relief only a few days at a time. Oral prednisone in doses of 20 mg daily helped temporarily, but then the pain returned.

When I had Barbara chart her baseline total pain score, she came back with a stunning 261! I determined that a priority was to get her off prednisone, but in the meantime I started her on cyclic estrogen and progestin. This allowed her to feel better almost immediately and to continue improving over the next few weeks. In two months her score was down to 110. This preliminary reduction of pain facilitates the patient's tolerance of the pains increased by the reduction-withdrawal of prednisone. When she reached the point at which one 5-mg tablet a day kept her within manageable bounds, I put her on the Diminished Directions Dosage of cyclic prednisone—10-5-5-5-5 mg for five days followed by six days off. This was admittedly difficult for Barbara at first, as she experienced severe pains on the days off that put her to bed. My advice was to ''tough it out.'' But once her bodily system had readapted, she did fine on the new lower levels of prednisone. Her pain score went down to 71, indicating that she was getting much more pain relief from the prednisone than before. In fact, Barbara came to feel so good that she made up her mind to go to college and start a career. And I am happy to report that she did just that . . . but she should return some time for additional arthritis help.

I would like to clearly point out that, when the large, continuous doses of Barbara's prednisone were replaced by the smaller, cyclic doses of prednisone, her pain scores became much smaller. 110 went down below 71, which suggests 35 percent less pain on 55 percent less prednisone. When her severe readjustment pains were over, she could detect the prednisone working for her. As I have observed in other patients with a similar pattern, the beneficial action of prednisone occurs when it is intermittently assisting hypothalamic-adrenal function rather than when it is constantly replacing and depressing hypothalamic-adrenal function. The evidence from Marcia and Barbara indicates that the five-day prednisone therapy recuperates the hypothalamus even if the total pain score is high, and then, when the prednisone is stopped, the hypothalamus works for as long as it can before again being suppressed by excessive inflammation.

Many physicians disagree with both the Microdose system and with the practice of letting the patient manage his or her own prednisone medication once the arthritis is under control. In my opinion, Microdose is the only prednisone route to achieving the goal we all share, which is long-term pain control for the patient. The strange practice of taking prednisone every day is just as ill-considered as it would be if, after your kitchen caught fire and the firemen put out the blaze, they continued to hose your house for days and weeks to come!

Managing Your Own Prednisone Therapy

These are instructions to help you get the maximum mileage out of your prednisone medication in a safe way:

Your first duty is to establish your baseline total pain score so that you can measure whether the prednisone is really helping or not. The Daily Pain Score and Pain Score Guide are described in Chapter 3.

Your second assignment is to take prednisone in the doses as outlined in the Prednisone Induction Guide, Table 1 Appendix C. The doses vary according to your body weight. Take each dosage for seven consecutive days, starting with the largest dose the first week and ending with the smallest dose the third week. With these three decreasing doses you will have a total of 21 days of uninterrupted medication. Take your pills each day between 7 and 8 A.M. to take maximum advantage of your body's circadian rhythm. If the total pain score should drop to nearly zero before the third week, advance your schedule to the third-week dose. Do not change your style of living during this time in order to avoid confusing the results: do not start or stop medications, do not go on food or drink binges, do not start or stop exercise classes and do not go on vacation. It is a rare patient who feels anything unusual while taking prednisone; but, if you do notice something worrisome, notify your doctor. If the improvement of your pain score is less than ten percent, it is probably not worthwhile continuing with prednisone, but proceed to the other therapies in this book. If the improvement in the pain score is ten percent or more, consider that the prednisone is of some value to you and you should progress to the next step of Microdose management.

Microdose management: If you feel that you no longer need your NSAIDs and other pain medications, you can now slowly reduce or discontinue them. Your new, lowered total pain score is now to be your new baseline score, so make record of it. Now turn to Appendix B for the Pain Guide for managing the Five-day Microdose Prednisone Treatment. Mark your baseline score. Take no more prednisone until the Pain Guide tells you to, and that is on the basis of your new total pain score. The pain scores listed under Act I tell you when to restart your prednisone if off medication five or more full days, and Act II tells you when to restart if off medication for four or fewer days. The strong hope is to be off five or more days. If you repeatedly restart before five days, it would be better to set your baseline a little higher.

Here's an example of how to proceed with the maintenance

phase. Please look at Table 2. Let's say that you took your last pill on Sunday when you arrived at a new baseline score of 10. On the following Friday morning, after four full days of no medication, your score has risen to 14. By the terms of Act II (four or fewer days), you must still wait to resume medication. By Saturday, when five full days without medication have passed and your score is still 14, Act I (five or more days) now says to start your prednisone, even though it is no higher than the day before. Do not restart your prednisone until your score reaches 14, even if a couple of weeks go by.

When it is time to act, be it Act I or Act II, go to the Five-Day Microdose Prednisone Treatment, Table 3 in Appendix C. This gives you your prednisone dosage schedule according to your weight. As in the earlier phase, take the medication between 7 and 8 a.m. The purpose of your prednisone dosage now is to push your elevated score back down to your new minimum baseline. If your score should decrease to the baseline before the five days have finished, and if you have taken the prednisone for at least three days, you may stop the prednisone right there. We want to be as stingy as possible with the use of prednisone. The minimum three days for medication is to provide recuperation for the hypothalamus. If you have not returned to baseline by the end of five days of medication, stop anyway! After stopping the prednisone, your pain score often drops still further, since that is a time when your hypothalamus may be working after its rest period. Medicating no more than five days and no less than three usually satisfies all needs.

If you should find that you are repeatedly restarting early according to Act II, it probably means that you should reset your baseline one number higher. Keep readjusting the baseline until there is a reasonable time pattern of five days off prednisone.

On the other hand, if you find that you are always going seven days or more with no medication before restarting your prednisone according to Act I and you are happy with the results, just stay the same and enjoy what you have gained. But, if you would like to have a lower baseline score, just reset your baseline one number smaller. Keep slowly adjusting until you find that both the time pattern and your comfort level meet your satisfaction. By the time you have stabilized, your average daily prednisone dosage will be no more than 3.5 mg, and usually much less.

A word of caution: Don't be tempted to keep pushing your prednisone intake too hard in order to attain an extra good score for today; in so doing, you will inevitably begin to trim back on the needed intervals of rest between taking medication, and can lose the benefits you have gained. Learn to be thankful for those benefits which can be both attained and maintained, be they large or small. Besides, as I describe in the remaining chapters, there are still other avenues of pain reduction to try if you have not yet reached your desired comfort level.

Many patients observe that, when they first start the Microdose prednisone therapy, they have considerable difficulty in going five days without medication; but, after they have treated themselves for a few months, the rest period of five days gradually increases in length spontaneously.

I hope you are persuaded of the value of the Microdose system and are willing to give it a try. If, however, you balk at so many calculations, here's a simpler, one-size-fits-all alternative. I call it the Diminished Directions Dosage or D-D-Dosage and it goes like this: Begin by going through the standard three-week induction. If you experience obvious improvement, go to a repeating schedule of prednisone five days on and six days off. Make the five-day dosage 10-5-5-5-5 mg, followed by a six-day respite. Under this regimen your average prednisone will be 2.7 mg daily. Still another schedule could be constructed around a 14-day cycle of five days on and nine days off, for a 2.1 mg daily average. This makes it possible for you to start on the same day of the week every second week. Remember that these averages are far below the theoretical toxic female borderline of 5.0. To be sure, these simplified systems cannot be as perfectly tailored to your body's individual needs as the first method I described, but they take less attention on the patient's part and work well enough in many cases. I also often use the D-D-Dosage when people have a high baseline, as with Barbara J.

Let me conclude Microdose with brief case histories of patients whose experiences substantiate my principles of prednisone therapy.

When I first met Andrea A #27, then aged 83, she had been living in a nursing home for seven months. Within only a month, Andrea told me, she had gone from being active in the normal chores of life on a farm to becoming wheelchair bound, all because of galloping rheumatoid arthritis. She complained of many painful and swollen joints, and I could see that the muscles of her arms and legs had become extremely weak from inactivity. Even with great effort she could now lift her foot no more than one inch off the floor, and neither aspirin nor the more potent NSAID Feldene had helped her noticeably. Cortisone shots in her right knee gave good relief, but only for a week at a time. We charted her baseline total pain score at 68.

I started Andrea on a prednisone induction, and within four hours of beginning therapy she was already feeling distinctly better, her pain reduced, her muscle power returning. When she charted her pain score at the end of the first 24 hours, she was amazed to find it at 27, and at the end of the three weeks' induction it was down to 5. Her knees were the last remaining site of pain, but her ankles and feet were still somewhat swollen. A month after her first visit, Andrea returned with a walker, having discarded her wheelchair. She walked slowly in slippers, but otherwise reasonably comfortably. We started a program of muscle conditioning to rebuild lost function, and when I checked her four weeks later she had replaced the walker with a cane. At three months she walked in with no assistance. As the swelling of her feet had now subsided, she was back in normal shoes. The pain in Andrea's knees has never gone away entirely, but she is satisfied with the enormous improvements that have been achieved and is able to go a month or more between Microdose prednisone treatments.

Loren Z #28 was a 50-year-old farmer's wife who suffered from severe rheumatoid arthritis for nine years. Loren's case typifies both modern physician abuse of prednisone and the conquering of her problem with other therapeutic measures. Many joints were swollen and painful for many years. Arthroscopy had been done for a ''torn knee cartilage,'' though she never injured her knee, and there were findings of severe arthritis. NSAIDs were of no value and the cancer medicine methotrexate produced only adverse reactions. She had been on prednisone for five years, and her dosage was 40 mg daily! Her menses ceased 17 years ago, and she experienced only a few hot flashes. Her weight was 220 pounds.

Loren's baseline score was way up at 181. The FED detected no food sensitivities. I prescribed Premarin 0.625 mg for days 1 through 24 and Provera 10 mg days 10 through 24 of the month. One month later she had lost 17 pounds and her pain score was down to 16. Loren then started decreasing her prednisone in steps down to 15 mg daily, but concomitantly there was a rise of the pain score to

60 to 80, with bursts up to 195. I then started her on spironolactone 100 mg daily. In 7 days the score was down to 32, in 21 days it was 8, and then in 56 days it went down to zero and stayed there. During this time the prednisone was slowly being decreased to 5 mg daily and then further decreased to 5 mg every three days. Loren's signal to take prednisone at that time was generalized stiffness rather than pain. At the present time she has no pain or stiffness at all, the swelling slowly left her knees completely, and she takes no prednisone unless there should be a rare pain from excess muscular activity.

Loren participated in a double-blind crossover study to verify that the pain relief experienced was medication-oriented rather than a placebo effect. On the two occasions when a placebo was used in place of the spironolactone, her pain score went up to 40 to 50 within the week, and there was a distinct collection of fluid in her knee joints. Otherwise her pain score was zero.

It took eleven months to wean Loren off the prednisone. The constant 40 mg dosage was excessive and abusive to her health. It did her no good, and I suspect that it aggravated her arthritis condition by depressing the protective functions of her hypothalamus and adrenal glands. Loren was lucky enough to avoid other specific side effects, but another young woman who recently consulted me developed cataracts within just one year of similar abuse with prednisone.

The very favorable decrease of over 100 points of pain for Loren in response to the progestin Provera suggest that it blocked the formation of the antigen which was being created by a native hapten progesterone. When the spironolactone was added, the score dropped to zero. It seems unlikely, if the spironolactone was merely supplementing the hapten control by the progestin, that there would be such a clear but gradual drop of about 70 more points of pain to zero over the course of 56 days. It seems more likely that the spironolactone was working in its capacity of altering steroidogenesis for removal of another portion of the antigen supply. The return of pain abruptly upon removal of the spironolactone during the experiment demonstrated that, although her bodily rheumatic manifestations certainly had healed and stayed healed for several months, the underlying system of antigen production had only been suppressed rather than being cured. That means that the medication must be maintained forever.

Linda V #29 came to see me at age 44. A farmer's wife and mother of four, she had developed rheumatoid arthritis suddenly seven years ago. Indocin helped her pains about 50 percent. Linda was very aware of a 75 percent exacerbation of her arthritis premenstrually, and this consisted of pain, tiredness, weakness and depression. She had gradually developed misalignment of her toes with hammertoes and toes overriding one another.

Her baseline score was 82. A cyclic estrogen plus progestin medication reduced the pain score to 70 and made an appreciable improvement in her menstrual discomfort. The FED brought the score down to 50, with caffeine being the apparent culprit. A prednisone induction now dropped the score to between 1 and 3 and is maintained there with Microdose prednisone. Her overriding toes are now spreading out properly and the hammertoes are slowly straightening out. She feels so good about herself that she has lost 35 pounds.

It seems unlikely that bone restructuring was involved in the changes of toe alignment. Subsiding of local tissue swelling and irritation certainly plays a part, but increased muscle strength and tone from better innervation and less inflammation probably plays a larger role. Prednisone is not an agent that makes toes go straight, but it is one of the agents that may control the rheumatic disease which makes the toes go crooked.

Patient Marion K #30 was a 24-year-old housewife whose rheumatoid arthritis had begun only two years previously. The pain had started in her shoulders and then spread rapidly all over her body. The bottoms of her feet hurt her so much that she could only hobble around on the outsides of her feet. She had developed prominent bunions, and her toes pointed downward and outward. Cortisone shots proved effective with shoulder and knee pains, but only briefly. None of the NSAIDs tried were good enough to give her better than a baseline score of 73.

I immediately introduced Marion to a prednisone induction, and over the next three weeks her symptoms receded until she had a new baseline score of 4. Her energy, strength and mood were also markedly improved. We found through the FED that caffeine was an irritating agent; with its removal her scores inched further down to 1, many times even zero. With her pain and inflammation gone, I told Marion to begin massaging and bending her toes toward their normal position and to practice standing and walking on the balls of her feet. After two months of this, she was able to walk painlessly, without a limp, and with her toes in normal alignment. The same excellent control persists more than four years later. I am unaware of such good foot results being reported before, and this is possibly because rheumatic inflammation has not been conquered so completely and so continuously.

Ida L #31 is yet another winner. When the 62-year-old Ida brought me her case, she said that for 14 years her combination of fibromyalgia and arthritis had resisted every effort of treatment. Indeed, her doctors had told her that, other than joining a psychological support group, she could not hope to relieve the fibromyalgia; for the arthritis, she had been offered NSAIDs and periodic cortisone shots in her back and elbow, with only mild, temporary relief.

Ida's baseline score was way up at 188, but with a prednisone induction we quickly brought it down to 61. Microdose prednisone maintenance brought it down further to 25. With the arthritis and fibromyalgia in retreat, we then took up the FED to bring her score down to 4 and frequently to zero. As is so often the case, coffee turned out to be the source of the allergic component of Ida's disease syndrome; by a process of elimination we discovered that drinking a single cup of regular coffee could make her score rise 10 or 15 points. Once the caffeine was gone from her system, the health problems that had plagued Ida for more than a decade essentially vanished, the supposedly "untreatable problem" of fibromyalgia included.

The experience of Chuck T #32 was also favorable, though its outcome was somewhat frustrating from a physician's point of view. Chuck came to me in his 35th year. A six-foot-four 205-pound sports director, he had been living with a certain amount of pain and stiffness in his neck and back since he was ten. About a dozen years ago it had become considerably more intrusive, and after seeing several specialists he was told that he had ankylosing spondylitis, a disease characterized by fusion of the vertebrae. By the time I saw Chuck, his rib cage had become so stiff that he had to do abdominal breathing, and to compensate for a markedly limited ability to turn his neck he usually had to turn his whole body. Two doses of Indocin daily had allowed him to moderate pain, but he had to carefully tend to the stomach distress this NSAID produced.

Chuck's initial baseline score was 10, and with prednisone it promptly dropped to 2. He stopped taking Indocin, and his stomach settled down. Pain flare-ups came with less and less frequency, and he was soon able to stabilize his prednisone intake so that he could go as long as 20 days between Microdose cycles, for an average prednisone dosage of 1.7 mg per day. The mobility of his neck has improved mildly. He sees no need for other dietary or medical intervention. Chuck is still teaching and playing tennis.

Anyone reading Chuck's story might reasonably assume that he represents one more example of a successful outcome through Microdose therapy. But I would like to have seen him go further, experimenting until the antigen(s) at the roots of his rheumatic problem had been identified and dealt with. My guess is that when the novelty of his new reduced pain state has worn off and when he gets older and his immune defenses diminish, he will want to return to follow the search for the causative antigen to its logical conclusion.

UNSCHEDULED DOSES OF PREDNISONE

I said earlier in this chapter that when you are on prednisone therapy, you should evaluate your total pain score upon arising each day to determine whether you need to take additional medication. This continues to be good practice. But now and then you may do something later in the same day that triggers an unusual and rapid inflammatory response; joints may become swollen and painful. Such flare-ups are usually due to food or an environmental factor, though strenuous activity can also be the culprit. We have discussed before that the sooner prednisone is given after a painful encounter, the less of a peak it will reach, the more rapidly the inflammatory response will go away, and the lower the dose needed for its ultimate control. For these reasons, I recommend that, when you experience a pain flare-up, you either initiate a new cycle of Microdose prednisone or supplement the dose taken earlier in the day. Be sure to record the new total pain score and the extra dose taken at the bottom of your Daily Pain Score. And if you have a good guess as to what may have precipitated your pain flare, write that down too. As soon as the flare-up has passed, return to your standard regimen and continue as before.

Once you recognize a recurring cause-and-effect for flare-ups, and you judge the trigger to be unavoidable or worth the pain, such as hoeing your garden, you can take a 5-mg tablet of prednisone as protective medicine before you start the activity. The objective is not just comfort, but to use less prednisone in the long run by aborting inflammation. But don't overdo it, or you will again face the failures caused by continuous prednisone medication.

MELATONIN, HORMONE HELPMATE

Based on my investigations, I conclude that the hormone melatonin plays an important role in treating rheumatic disease. Melatonin is a chemical secreted principally in the pineal gland, a small cone-shaped body deep within the mid-portion of your brain; lesser amounts of melatonin are also made in your intestines. The hormone is produced mostly in the nighttime phase of the body's circadian rhythm. Though the way this occurs is not entirely known, it appears to be somehow related to the amount of light entering the eye; the more light, the less melatonin and vice versa. As the age of 40 approaches, melatonin production decreases rather steeply; so by 45 your production may be only half of what it was in youth; and it continues to slow as age advances.

Melatonin supplements are sold over the counter in drug stores and natural health food stores. Reportedly it enhances sleep. Large, prolonged overdosage has no reported side effects. It is a strong antioxidant with a special ability to protect your DNA. As an immune-system stimulant, this hormone supplement is generally labeled with a warning against using it in the presence of any autoimmune disease, such as rheumatoid arthritis. But I take the opposite position; contrary to standard practice, which favors the suppression of the immune system to reduce antibody response, my therapeutic approach specifically calls for stimulation of the immune system. And the experience of my arthritis patients suggests that I am right. I recommend melatonin supplements daily, 1 to 5 mg just before bedtime. My wife and I both take it and we each experienced mildly better rheumatic comfort and sleep. Melatonin will not cure you, but it has a reasonable chance for making your life a little bit better in a simple, natural way. Do not, however, take it without monitoring your daily total pain score. Even with so generally benign a substance as melatonin, there is always the one-in-a-million possibility that you will have an unexpected adverse effect and need to recognize it for what it is.

REMEMBER

1. Prednisone, when used properly, has essentially no serious side effects; used improperly, however, it can have very negative consequences in treating arthritis.

2. Microdose prednisone gives far better long-term pain relief than standard prednisone therapy.
3. Microdose prednisone often helps all types of rheumatic disease, including fibromyalgia, when followed carefully.
4. A Diminished-Directions-Dosage system simplifies management in some cases.
5. I believe that the daily administration of prednisone for arthritis is detrimental and contraindicated.
6. Melatonin can help rheumatic disease by being an antioxidant, by enhancing the immune system, and by enhancing sleep.
7. Even huge doses of melatonin have been found to have no harmful effects. The usual dosage of melatonin is 1 to 5 mg taken at bedtime.

8

Spironolactone

THE DIURETIC WITH A DIFFERENCE

SPIRONOLACTONE IS my favorite personal arthritis medication, because it played a major part in bringing me back from the despair and pain of my own osteoarthritis some years ago. With spironolactone I was able to go a long way toward regaining my former levels of comfort and function, and I have since found the drug to be effective for many other people with various types of arthritis. It is not, however, for everyone, as I will explain later.

Spironolactone is a chemical derivative of the steroid female sex hormone progesterone. Rejiggered in the laboratory, the manmade molecule has many of the properties common to conventional diuretics or "water pills," with the added feature that it does not deplete the body's stores of essential potassium in the process of removing other salts. This feature makes spironolactone a good choice in treating many cases of high blood pressure and in removing the excess fluids associated with edema conditions, such as ankle swelling and heart failure.

Spironolactone is the most frequently used blood pressure controlling medication in modern countries, such as in Japan and France, though it is somewhat less favored for this purpose in the U.S.A. There are three established mechanisms by which spironolactone works to control blood pressure. First is its diuretic action. Second, it acts as a calcium channel blocker. That means it keeps calcium inside the smooth muscle cells of your blood vessels to keep them relaxed. Third, in competition with the steroid hormone aldosterone, it controls sodium release from smooth muscle cell membranes for additional blood vessel relaxation. Spironolactone is sometimes taken in combination with other thiazide diuretics in order to counteract the low potassium which the thiazides tend to produce.

In addition, spironolactone can be used as a strong partner of allopurinol to control gout (as we'll see with patients JL #38 and BJ #39 in the next chapter).

Like progesterone, spironolactone has also been found to have some hormonal activity. It is through this function, rather than as an analgesic or anti-inflammatory agent, which spironolactone is not, that I believe this medication has a positive effect on rheumatic disease. One mechanism of function which I propose is that spironolactone's steroid shape allows it to attach to the same hormonal receptor sites that antigenic hormones compete for, and in covering those sites before the antigen can, it blocks their arthritis-causing action. Unable to latch onto key receptors, the antigens simply do not trigger an arthritic response. This same hormonal activity is probably the source of some other effects that have been noted with spironolactone; for example, the drug has been known to decrease hair growth on the face, chest and arms by blocking androgen receptors; and to cause temporary breast enlargement and tenderness. It is also well established that spironolactone alters steroidogenesis (hormone manufacture) in the ovaries, testicles and adrenal glands, and there is clear evidence that this change is in both quality and quantity (Loriaux 1976, Serafini and Lobo 1985). This alteration can possibly diminish or remove steroid chemicals considered to be alien by the immune system.

Because spironolactone does not deplete potassium in the process of being a diuretic, it is important that anyone taking it not take extra potassium at the same time. This means avoiding not only potassium salts, but also such potassium buildup medicines as triamterene (Dyrenium), amiloride (Moduretic), and any of the angiotensin-converting enzyme (ACE) inhibitors, and the anti-inflammatory drug Indocin. I also recommend caution in prescribing spironolactone for people with a prolonged history of hypertension and diabetes mellitus, and for anyone who is either of an advanced age or who has used high-dose NSAIDs over a prolonged period, on the presumption that their kidneys may have sustained some damage. In such cases I always order a blood screening beforehand for the levels of potassium and creatinine for safety, though I have yet to find one in trouble. If the test indicates that the kidneys are not functioning adequately, I would steer away from the drug. Spironolactone is contraindicated for persons with significantly impaired kidney function, which in practicality is uncommonly encountered.

So long as these exceptions are granted, spironolactone can be safely used in arthritis treatment. Studies involving many tens of thousands of patients taking spironolactone indicate no serious side effects. Occasional breast tenderness and some nighttime leg muscle cramps have been the most serious problems reported by my patients. And the beneficial effects of spironolactone are real, not placebo-derived, as I was able to demonstrate several years ago in a double-blind, crossover clinical trial involving a representative sample of spironolactone patients. I presented the results at the Fifth Interscience World Conference on Inflammation in Geneva, Switzerland in 1993.

My Clinical Use of Spironolactone

As I have said before, I do not differentiate among the variously-named types of arthritis in devising treatment for my patients. Almost everyone with arthritis can potentially benefit from spironolactone, those with damaged kidneys being the primary exception.

Spironolactone is available in both generic and proprietary forms. As the generics, which are produced in 25-mg tablets, work extremely well, I have found no need to procure the more expensive name brand, Aldactone. The recommended dosage is based on the patient's weight, using the formula of 1 mg per pound per day. To show how that works out, let's suppose your weight is 145 pounds; your dose is then 125 mg, 150 mg being a little excessive. I recommend using an even somewhat smaller dose if it does a good job. For myself, I use 100 mg daily instead of the 125 mg to which I am "entitled." The best time to take spironolactone is in the morning, either with or without a meal. After the first few days, the diuretic effect becomes barely noticeable, but it is still more convenient to have even a mild diuretic effect during waking hours than when you want to sleep.

The first step in determining whether spironolactone is of any benefit to you is to establish your baseline total pain score. You then take spironolactone every day while you monitor your pain score for six weeks, changing nothing else in your routine for the time being. Do not start or stop any other medicine, do not go on any wild eating or drinking binges, do not start or stop any exercise programs, and do not go on vacation, because these factors might give you skewed results. If there is no decrease in your total pain score in six weeks, you conclude that spironolactone is of no value for you and stop taking it. In order for you to respond to spironolactone, you must have had from the beginning a reaction or sensitivity to your own hormones.

If, however, you do chart a decrease in your total pain score over the six weeks, you can reasonably conclude that some benefit is being obtained from the spironolactone. At that point, you may want to try a slightly smaller dose, say one less tablet, to see if it still does a good job for you. Once you have found an optimal dose, plan to stay on it forever. Don't fret about occasional lapses, like forgetting a day or taking a tablet too many: with spironolactone you can afford to make mistakes without detriment, but if you make a big one, like skipping three to six days for example, your body will protest with enough aches and pains to get you back on the ball!

Even after you achieve that first drop in pain score at the end of the first six weeks, you may get still more downward movement, but don't expect spironolactone alone to take you to zero unless you are very lucky. Look for some of the other therapeutic measures I describe to take you the remaining distance.

I'd like to return now to the story of Lucy J #3, described in some detail in Chapter 4, because she is such an excellent teaching example. You will remember that Lucy came to me for rheumatoid arthritis which had developed about ten years earlier when Lucy was in her fifties. She also reported that she was being treated for high blood pressure, which was 172/92 under the influence of ACE inhibitors. Lucy also told me that when NSAIDs had given her no relief, her rheumatologist had tried multiple cortisone injections. When these too proved unsatisfactory, he referred her to an orthopedic surgeon who examined both knees by arthroscopy. The orthopedist by looking into the joint could find no clear evidence of arthritis damage nor could he come up with any reliable means of symptomatic relief.

I began treatment as always by establishing Lucy's baseline total pain score. You may remember that with prednisone induction we brought her score from 117 down to 95, and went on with the aid of the FED to lower the score further to 70, though at times it would bounce back up to 107. Lucy turned out to have several allergies including wheat, oats and yeast, which are silent partners in many compound foods, and consequently difficult to screen out entirely. When she was stabilized again, I decided it was time to introduce spironolactone daily, an event that caused me to discontinue further use of the ACE inhibitor that she had been taking for her blood pressure.

On a regimen of 100 mg spironolactone daily, Lucy's score dropped spectacularly to zero! Her blood pressure went down to 142/80. Taking the medication did not guarantee her freedom from pain; on occasions when she inadvertently ate wheat, her score would rise to 40 within the day and take about five days to subside again. But the discomfort she felt on those occasions was still a far cry from where she had been without spironolactone. Interestingly, the distribution of her joint pains and their aching nature were essentially identical, no matter whether triggered by a food allergen or by the endogenous hormones to which Lucy was evidently sensitized. The only real difference was in the intensity, which expressed itself in the total pain score. In other words, it was the summation of immune complexes (food and hormones) that determined both the presence and intensity of her rheumatic disease.

The fact that diet, not spironolactone, was the only way to inhibit the antigenic effect of wheat, while spironolactone was 100 percent successful in blocking the inflammatory effect of some natural hormone in Lucy's body, makes it clear that spironolactone works not on inflammation directly, but on the immune complexes that precede inflammation. By sorting out these multiple causes and multiple "cures," we were able to produce a total turnaround of Lucy's health status.

I informed Lucy that the blood test showed she was on the borderline for spironolactone. I explained that, should her kidneys get worse, we might have to stop the spironolactone to prevent her collecting too much potassium, which in turn could lead to a sudden heart standstill and death. She explained that I would *never* get the medicine away from her, because she would far rather die such an early, *beautiful* heart death than ever return to the worthless, miserable existence with arthritis pain!

Similarly, my patient Gina P #33 got her health and her life back with the help of spironolactone. When Gina came to me for her first appointment, she was 41 years old and a struggling mother with two teenage children. She had lived with severe rheumatoid arthritis since the age of 12, which was coincidentally the onset of her periods. Her physician had prescribed the corticosteroid prednisone 7.5 mg daily to modify her symptoms. At age 21 and shortly after marrying, Gina stopped her medication in preparation for becoming pregnant. During pregnancy she was surprised and thrilled to note that her rheumatic symptoms largely disappeared, even though her bony joints had already undergone many distinct changes that evidenced a history of arthritis. And no sooner had she given birth than her rheumatic problems returned with greater severity than before. Her physician increased her prednisone intake to 10 mg daily as needed. Then, following the birth of her second child when Gina was 25, her diagnosis of rheumatoid arthritis was changed to systemic lupus erythematosus, based on a positive blood cell test. For the next 15 years she took daily maintenance doses of prednisone 5 to 10 mg, and with her immune system as suppressed as it was, she eventually began having episodes of life-threatening bacteremia (bacteria growing in her bloodstream) about every month or two. No sooner was Gina out of the hospital from one bacteremia than she was back in for another. Her muscles were chronically sore and her joints painful, red, swollen, stiff and progressively deformed.

It was at this point that Gina, feeling her life severely threatened, came to me hoping for some new approach. My medical instinct led me to begin by placing her on spironolactone 100 mg daily together with 400 I.U. of vitamin E daily to counter some of her inflammation. Within ten days Gina experienced marked relief of her rheumatic symptoms to the point that she was more comfortable than at any time in memory. The joint redness and pain that had been with her so long subsided, and the swelling that had plagued her disappeared so that she could see her knuckles for the first time in many years. As soon as I was satisfied that the lupus was in retreat, I began to reduce her prednisone slowly, until she was able to stop taking it entirely at the end of 12 weeks. As this was the first time I had ever attempted to take a patient off prednisone, I proceeded with great caution, decreasing dosage by 1 mg every two weeks. Knowing what I know now, I might accomplish the same task in a much shorter time.

Gina suffered no adverse effects from prednisone withdrawal and was soon feeling consistently so well with no pain that she took a full-time factory job. Her remarkable improvement was confirmed in a routine checkup two years later when she was age 43. She was vigorous, healthy and happy! When she was very sick, her antibody titer was 1:300, and now, when she was perfectly well, it was 1:1,200!! Only the blood test was sick!

Gina's story does not end there, however. Shortly after my last checking her, she caught a cold which came on with sufficient energy that she took herself to the emergency room for treatment. When the physician who saw her learned that she had been diagnosed with lupus and was not on prednisone, a rheumatologist was called in on the case, and Gina was put in the hospital immediately. Following standard protocols, the rheumatologist ordered the spironolactone stopped and prednisone 10 mg was restarted. By the time Gina was released from the hospital one week later, she had been persuaded to return to her old prednisone-based treatment. Sadly, her old symptoms returned with a vengeance within a month, and soon she was unable to work. It was not long before Gina was suffering from extreme hypertension, cardiac failure, recurrent infections, and kidney and liver failure. She died at age 44.

It is interesting and surprising to observe in Gina that the adrenal gland and hypothalamus, which had been theoretically fully suppressed by 5 to 10 mg prednisone daily for thirty years, were able to return to apparently normal function in less than twelve weeks' time and to continue functioning normally for the subsequent two years in excellent health on the spironolactone alone—until the prednisone was restarted. The total pain score of zero means that the hypothalamic, pituitary and adrenal glands must be working very properly.

Patient Loren Z #28 took prednisone for five years with doses up to 40 mg, and it took her 11 months with moderate symptoms to get off prednisone. Gina P #33 was on prednisone with doses 5 to 10 mg for 30 years, and it took her only three months to get off easily without symptoms of withdrawal. Whether the time difference for weaning depends more upon the strength of dose or the length of taking it, I do not know. Possibly it is just individual differences. It seems that regardless of how long the hypothalamus, pituitary and adrenals have been turned off or suppressed, they have the potential for returning to apparently normal function (Paris 1961).

I believe that Gina would almost certainly be alive today if she had continued to control her autoimmune disease with spironolactone, as it had so clearly demonstrated it could. But she fell victim to medical tradition and an unwillingness to trust her own experience when faced with the weighty opinions of so many contrary authorities. I believe that the poor prognosis for lupus is at least partly a result of the adverse effects of constant prednisone administration.

I have had a few other patients with the diagnosis of lupus erythematosus come to my office for advice. Most have been so severely frightened by the dire prognoses given by their rheumatologists that they have been unwilling to try a therapy, even briefly, that does not have the positive consensus of physicians. By so doing, they committed themselves to failure!

One happy exception who left the ranks of standard medicine is Jessie W #34. Diagnosed with lupus, she had the courage to tarry with me while we tried to find the genesis of her lupus. Jessie now has 95 percent control of her disease, with spironolactone being an important part of her successful regimen.

Gina's and Jessie's very different lupus outcomes show once again how important it is for every patient to learn about their own individual condition, to consider the logic and potentials of the various therapies offered by their doctors, and finally to become actively engaged in determining how to proceed. As I tell each of my patients, and I say to you, "Don't take another person's advice as the final word without thinking for yourself on what you must do to get better. This is *your* life!"

ADDITIONAL TALES OF SUCCESS

In concluding this chapter on spironolactone, I will cite a couple of additional cases that were successfully treated by using this remarkable manmade medication in a way not originally anticipated by its developers.

Polly O'B #35 was a 50-year-old nurse when I first saw her in 1992. She had experienced osteoarthritis pains for the previous seventeen years, the discomfort becoming especially pronounced in the past two years. Treatment for Polly had ranged from NSAIDs (only mildly helpful) to chiropractic (slightly better). She had also undergone a hysterectomy to reduce the pain associated with endometriosis. She was regularly taking thiazides and ACE inhibitors for hypertension that ranged around 170/100 with full medication. Not long before she came to see me, her previous doctor had given her a comprehensive examination, including blood tests, to evaluate her rheumatic status. When all features of the examination and blood tests had come back essentially normal, Polly's doctor concluded that she did not have arthritis and to leave well enough alone!

I found Polly's baseline total pain score to be 70. I began treating her with a prednisone induction, and this promptly brought her score down to 15. Using the FED, I isolated caffeine and cantaloupe as reactive food factors, and brought the score down further to 5. As Polly discontinued her thiazide and ACE inhibitors, I started her on spironolactone 100 mg daily. This took her down one last notch until she hovered between zero and 1. Her blood pressure came to within normal limits, stabilizing around 146/86. Nowadays Polly needs prednisone only for occasional flare-ups of pain. Polly's multistage progress toward freedom from pain can be explained in the following way: prednisone was used initially to neutralize the immune complexes that were already collecting at various sites in her body; elimination of specific reactive foods reduced the number of immune complexes; spironolactone reduced the immune complexes nearly to zero, so she rarely needed any more prednisone.

Polly's case can be taken as an informative tale for those doctors who rely too heavily on laboratory tests and too little on their patients' words in making difficult diagnoses. When Polly's original physician told her that, because her tests revealed nothing abnormal, there was nothing more to do for her pains, he abdicated his medical responsibility. I believe that many medical tests end up being more of a hindrance than a help to doctors, because they get in the way of medical intuition and experience, which are critical to getting to the heart of many health problems.

Carol Z #36 also supports this point. When Carol came to see me, she was a 38-year-old divorced mother of four. As the sole owner and manager of a working farm, she did the strenuous work of running the trucks and huge combine machines herself. But she was having a hard time keeping up with the demands of her life. Back pains that had troubled her since the age of 16 had in the last four years become worse, spreading as well to her hips and feet. A family physician had told her that the pains were caused by osteoarthritis and had first recommended NSAIDs and later cortisone shots, but to no avail. Surgical replacement of her right hip was an option that was recommended shortly before she came to see me. During our first meeting Carol also reported severe problems with menstrual bleeding and said that she often felt overheated, causing her to sweat profusely, often in the middle of the night. Carol also had known food allergies to strawberries and tomatoes and was lactose intolerant. Clearly, there was a lot of tumult going on in Carol's system, and it was my job to sort out the parts and see what could be done to get her some relief.

First, we established Carol's baseline total pain score, which turned out to be 41. Next I put her on cyclic estrogen and progestin, and these took care of her menstrual problems, but did not change her arthritis pain score or the hot feelings. I also recommended that she be more careful in avoiding her reactive foods and foods containing milk and milk by-products. We then moved on to prednisone induction, which brought her score down to 16, except during the week before her period began, when it would rise up again. Finally, when she was more or less stabilized, I prescribed spironolactone 100 mg daily. This not only brought a halt to her hot feelings and night sweats, but lowered her pain score to a steady 3. From that time on, Carol felt in charge of her life and her farm, and she has remained so in the years since. Ask her what she thinks about having her hip replaced surgically and she will tell you that such an idea now seems ridiculous. As is often the case, I cannot tell you exactly how spironolactone accomplished its particular miracles in restoring Carol's health, but she recognizes its worth and looks forward to taking it indefinitely as a key player in her transformation. It just might be important in your recovery too!

Joel S #37 was a 75-year-old farmer when he came to see me about his osteoarthritis, which had been present for 25 years. Recently his hands and fingers had become so painful and swollen that he could not use them. His lifelong friend and doctor prescribed an ACE inhibitor for his hypertension and nearly valueless NSAIDs for his pain.

When Joel came to visit me, his initial blood pressure was 170/90 and his baseline pain score was 56. Spironolactone 100 mg daily was prescribed as the ACE inhibitor was discontinued. He was very pleased that in one month the pain score was 10 and after three months it was 5. His blood pressure went down to 142/84. His family doctor and friend did not like the spironolactone, so angrily ordered it stopped, and if Joel didn't comply, he would never speak to him again! As a result of stopping the spironolactone, all the pain returned to completely incapacitate him again. After consulting with me about his personal problem, Joel again obtained great relief from the spironolactone in spite of his doctor-"friend's" threats!

REMEMBER

1. Spironolactone is a steroid hormone derivative that has the potential for blocking other antigenic hormones. It alters steroid construction in adrenals, ovaries and testes to hopefully make them less antigenic.
2. Spironolactone controls blood pressure by salt reduction, water reduction, calcium channel blocking and smooth muscle relaxation.
3. Spironolactone appears to be effective in treating all types of rheumatic disease.
4. With the exception of patients with poor kidney function and those on potassium-saving medications, spironolactone is a safe medication without significant side effects.
5. Spironolactone is effective in rheumatic disease, not by being directly anti-inflammatory or analgesic, but by inhibiting the formation of immune complexes that ultimately produce the inflammation.

9

Gout, Gouty Arthritis and Pseudo-Gout

IT AIN'T WHAT IT USED TO BE

GOUT IS an intermittent but excruciatingly painful type of arthritis. For centuries it was unfairly blamed on gluttony and voluptuous living, and called "the king of disease and the disease of kings," because it afflicted so many of Europe's royal personages, who were, coincidentally, prone to excesses in their behavior. But we now know that the disease is based on a defect in metabolism, often passed on from one generation to the next. Gout usually appears when the body manufactures excess uric acid, a waste product, and when the kidneys are unable to excrete all that is made into the urine. High levels of the uric acid therefore accumulate in the blood, then precipitate out, forming needle-like crystals that collect in joints and their membranous interfaces like so many grains of sand. As the discussion that follows indicates, there are enough different theories about the fundamental causes of gout and how it should be controlled to suggest that the correct answers are yet to be found. But I have my own good ideas, and I have had enough therapeutic success in treating gout and gouty arthritis in my own contrarian way to have no hesitation sharing the thoughts and my casebook with you.

SOME TEXTBOOK THEORY

Gout troubles about 2,000,000 Americans, men more frequently than women, and starting most often after the age of thirty in men and after the menopause in women. Being overweight also seems to be associated with gout, with about half of gout sufferers carrying 15 percent excess pounds or more. Patients with acute and chronic gout are statistically more likely than average to have high blood pressure, diabetes and hardening of the arteries.

Uric acid is a normal metabolite, but people with gout make an excessive amount of uric acid because of faulty enzyme action. Associated with this is an increased level of uric acid in the blood. When the blood tests over 6.8, it is considered to be supersaturated, so irritating crystals will tend to form. Of all those people with an elevated uric acid, only 30 percent will develop gout, and 10 percent of those with gout have normal blood uric acid levels.

A significant minority also have kidney problems ranging from uric acid kidney stones to significant kidney malfunction. The kidney malfunction may be the result of metabolic overproduction of uric acid at another site, delivering more uric acid to the kidneys than even healthy kidneys can handle, or it may arise from some inflammatory problem in the kidneys that inhibits normal functioning. In either case, the organs chiefly responsible for filtering blood and secreting waste products struggle to process superconcentrated, supersaturated solutions of uric acid with limited success. Tiny uric acid crystals may adhere to one another, clogging the tubular channels that normally transport the kidneys' waste products, or slowly form stones that later pass down the urinary tract causing excruciating, if short-term, mechanical pain.

Some of the uric acid crystals collect in joints, most typically at the base of the big toe, but also in the knees and hands. A belief long held about gout is that it occurs in the big toes and fingers because they are in a colder part of the body, thereby enhancing the potential for precipitation of the crystals. But if cold were truly a basic feature of crystallization, then acute attacks would occur when sportsmen are outdoors in winter for so many hours; in fact, attacks are more likely to occur in the middle of the night in a nice warm bed.

Sometimes additional crystals originate in softer tissues to form characteristic nodules or deposits under the skin called tophi. Tophi may appear on the outer surfaces of elbows, hands, knees, feet and in the cartilage of the earlobes. They range up to about three centimeters in size, have variable tenderness, and typically consist of a core of uric acid crystals around which are concentric rings of immune cells. A tophus may ulcerate and discharge chalky material from the skin's surface or into the joint spaces. Very small tophi, called microtophi, are also formed in large numbers in the synovial membranes of the joints. If there is no accompanying inflammation, the freed crystals will be inactive and probably slowly dissolve away to nothingness.

Symptoms of gouty arthritis vary. In some patients, crystals in the joints can cause acute attacks of very severe joint inflammation, swelling, pain and fever. An acute attack of gout typically peaks in 24 to 48 hours and then subsides within a week to ten days, though it may last several weeks if not treated. Sometimes the toe is so exquisitely tender that even the touch of bed sheets causes intolerable pain. (This kind of extreme skin sensitivity is sometimes found in rheumatoid arthritis as well.) In other patients the crystals produce a chronic low-level discomfort that mimics osteoarthritis. Still other patients tolerate the crystals well, and have a complete lack of symptoms. The uric acid crystals that form in and around the joint reputedly inflame the surrounding tissues to produce arthritis. White blood cells respond to the crystal irritation and start attacking the crystals; but when they attempt to do so, they initiate a complicated chemical process that contributes yet more inflammation, with the result that the body's first line of defense often does more harm than good in the short run. Colchicine, a powerful drug made from the flower of the autumn crocus, is frequently used to treat these painful acute episodes, and it is remarkably effective. What is remarkable about colchicine is that it brings relief even though the offending uric acid crystals remain, now rendered nonirritating, even after the inflammation has subsided completely. It is also worth noting that the same uric acid crystals can be found in many normal joints, and there again they produce no joint pains.

How can this be? you ask, as I once did. The most logical explanation is that under normal circumstances a type of protein called an apoprotein covers the electrochemically charged crystals to render them inactive. But where faulty metabolism exists, the apoprotein coverings can be displaced by some other chemical substance and the crystal is suddenly made highly reactive to white cells (Ortiz-Bravo et al. 1993). What causes or controls the coating of the crystals to be displaced is not known by rheumatologists.

We know that the metabolic error in gout is controlled by genetic factors. But we do not yet know why this problem doesn't reveal itself in youth, though it has been postulated that the kidney clearance of uric acid in the young is great enough to overcome excessive production. We also do not know why it appears more often and earlier in males than females, how the menopause in particular affects the usual startup time for women, or what part obesity may contribute to the puzzle, though it may be something as simple as the fact that excess weight increases mechanical pressure on already vulnerable joints.

One thing we know about gout is that it is sometimes responsive to dietary changes. Some gout sufferers can reduce the frequency and severity of attacks by avoiding purine-rich foods such as peas, beans, sardines, anchovies, scallops and organ meats, all of which naturally produce large amounts of uric acid during the metabolic processing. However, avoidance of such foods has little impact on those gout sufferers whose blood uric acid levels are consistently high. We also know that alcohol interferes with uric acid metabolism, which would be enough to explain why excessive consumption can make gout worse. But there is also recent research indicating that alcohol inhibits the immune system. Alcohol is, incidentally, listed in the high-risk Class V in my Table of Food Classification.

As alcohol is a negative, drinking lots of water to flush the kidneys is a strong positive; otherwise, the tiny uric acid crystals that form in the kidneys can either cause blockages or group together to form kidney stones. Severe kidney damage used to be a common accompaniment of gouty arthritis, but better managing techniques seem to have nearly eliminated that severe problem from our list of worries.

Medical reports indicate that gout is accentuated by the presence of certain other medicines. One area of concern is diuretic medications, especially the thiazides, which lower blood pressure by promoting the formation and release of extra amounts of urine and salt. As high blood pressure and gout are sometimes companion disorders, special attention must be paid in prescribing for this group of individuals. Aspirin has also been found occasionally to precipitate an acute attack of gouty arthritis or even exacerbate an existing attack. For complicated reasons, aspirin up to 2 grams per day decreases kidney uric acid clearance, while doses over 2 g per day markedly increase kidney uric acid excretion. This indicates that if you use aspirin at all (I don't recommend it), use it in doses that add up to more than 2 g a day.

Gout medication is recommended only to patients who have had symptomatic problems with uric acid. Therapy typically consists of three agents: colchicine, which is used solely for control of acute attacks; and two types of medicines, probenecid and allopurinol, that lower uric acid levels in different ways.

The Roles of Probenecid and Allopurinol

Probenecid is classified as a uricosuric agent, or one that causes the kidneys to excrete double their usual amount of uric acid. Joints may become more comfortable and tophi may shrink under a continuing regimen of probenecid, but overproduction of uric acid remains unchanged. The benefits come about as the result of blood levels of uric acid being lowered and less of it precipitating in the joints. Probenecid is sometimes used for individuals who have only small amounts of uric acid in the urine. Typical dosage of probenecid is 0.5 g four times daily, but it will need adjustments by your doctor. The duration of treatment is lifelong. A few patients experience stomach distress or rash, but the great majority tolerate it well.

Allopurinol is usually preferred for patients whose urine contains large amounts of uric acid. The drug works by actually inhibiting the enzyme that produces uric acid in the first place; with less uric acid produced, there is less to spill over into the joints to cause gout, and there is less to form kidney crystals. As the allopurinol takes effect, the tissue cells become more healthy. The healthier tissues may still become irritated, but not as severely or as frequently as before the allopurinol therapy. Some crystals may just dissolve away from tophi and joints.

The dosage of allopurinol, which is adjusted to the severity of the symptoms, is usually 200 to 600 mg a day, with a maximum of 800 mg. Such doses, along with decreasing the frequency and intensity of gouty attacks in most patients, can also diminish existing tophi and lessen the likelihood of uric acid kidney stones. Though a restrictive diet can be somewhat relaxed while taking allopurinol, I urge my patients to avoid high-purine foods as much as possible to avoid becoming entirely dependent on the medication, which can have side effects of its own. It is advised that allopurinol shouldn't be started at the time of an acute flare-up, because it can actually make symptoms worse. And it is also not recommended for people whose gout occurs only infrequently.

PSEUDO-GOUT

Mimicking aspects of classic gout is another joint-related medical condition known as pseudo-gout. Pseudo-gout is a condition also characterized by acute inflammation, but due to the accumulation of calcium crystals rather than uric acid crystals. The calcium crystals most commonly form in the larger joints, primarily the knees and wrists, rather than the big toes, and are more likely to develop after the age of 60. Psuedo-gout crystals are also associated with osteoarthritis, and calcium and uric acid crystals can occur together in the same patient and in the same joint, which can be very painful indeed.

No known medication can stop the formation of calcium joint crystals to prevent pseudo-gout, but NSAIDs and aspirin can ease the pain. Colchicine is sometimes used to provide symptomatic relief of acute pseudo-gout pain.

CONTROVERSIES AND MY NEW THEORIES

All the preceding information is as modern science sees it. I agree with most of the given facts and theories, but some of them I will soon carefully explain to you by evidence and by logic to be either incomplete or incorrect. I will first discuss four gouty arthritis cases I have treated in my new fashion so that you can see the improved results in action, and then I will discuss in detail why my new theories and therapies work so much better.

Julie L #38 was a 43-year-old mother of two when she first came to see me. She was severely overweight—at five feet six she weighed 269 pounds—and severely hobbled by arthritis-type pain. Her condition, which started ten years before, had been diagnosed by her first doctor as ordinary osteoarthritis, but had failed to respond to several measures of conventional arthritis therapy. When Julie's physician had finally tried allopurinol and found it to work well, he concluded that she had classic gout, and treated her accordingly, with some success.

But six years after her symptoms began, Julie and her family moved to another state. Her new doctor, after going over all her records and performing his own examination, disagreed with the diagnosis of gout. He found, as I would later confirm, that she had normal levels of uric acid in her blood. He took Julie off allopurinol and put her on NSAIDs. Julie's condition soon worsened, her disability gradually increasing to the point of barely being able to walk into his office. Each year for four years, when Julie suggested that they resume allopurinol, her physician repeated his firm belief that allopurinol was appropriate only for treating gout, a disease she did not have! In four years he never read a text to obtain the whole truth!

Following our first meeting, Julie took a week to work out her baseline total pain score, and reported back that she averaged 32. I first prescribed spironolactone 100 mg daily for her, because I felt that it was safer medicine than the allopurinol. In six weeks her score was down to 8. She still had some pains and burning numbness in her right toes, which previously had been somewhat better controlled by the allopurinol. I then prescribed a minimal dosage of allopurinol

100 mg daily as a starter. Her pains and numbness essentially disappeared. With further tinkering, Julie was able to cut back on the allopurinol until she was maintaining herself pain free on a combination of daily 100 mg spironolactone and 100 mg allopurinol every second day. She continues this regimen today. She has occasional flare-ups of pain, indistinguishable from those of classic gout, but they occur mildly with monthly regularity at the time of her ovulation or when she engages in some unusual physical exercise. At that time a short dose of Microdose prednisone quickly returns her to no pain.

It is somewhat difficult to defend Julie's initial diagnosis of gout, given that her uric acid levels were within normal limits, but her very satisfactory response to allopurinol with her first doctor, as well as under my care, and the reversals of health she experienced when off it, certainly bespeak some metabolic error in the area of uric acid. It suggests that her kidneys had escaped the usual damage associated with gout, and this favorable circumstance had allowed for normal uric acid excretion. Lupus patients also demonstrate great variability in the degree of their renal involvement.

Pharmaceutical guidelines tell us that the minimal effective dose of allopurinol is 100 to 200 mg daily; yet Julie, at the substantial weight of 269 pounds, is able to do well on an average of 50 mg daily. This suggests to me that there may be some beneficial, synergistic, metabolic effect of the combination of spironolactone and allopurinol, each one boosting the effectiveness of the other.

Please note that the joint pain which flared up regularly during ovulation was identical to her gout pain, suggesting that her ovulatory hormones were reproducing the exact conditions of gouty arthritis. It is very unlikely that uric acid crystals would reactivate themselves coincidentally with every ovulation. One could alternately propose that she has a combination of diseases, but I find it more logical to start with the premise that she has but one basic disease process, a periodic excess of immune complexes, originating at least in part from ovarian progesterone, which produces the one entity of gouty arthritis. One thing remains certain: because of unconventional therapy, Julie's life has changed dramatically for the better.

I must admit that I cannot tell you exactly how Julie L, with a very normal uric acid, was improved 75 percent by spironolactone and then the other 25 percent by allopurinol—whether by favorably altering local tissue uric acid metabolism, by controlling immune complexes, or perhaps a combination of both processes.

My next report is about Bart J #39, who at age 71 had been living with a diagnosis of gouty arthritis for more than ten years. Bart had taken allopurinol for his gout and the NSAID indomethacin constantly and at maximum dosage for the pain. His blood uric acid was 10.4, considerably above normal.

When Bart came to see me, his baseline total pain score was 11. I prescribed spironolactone 100 mg daily in addition to his allopurinol. After only one month of spironolactone, Bart's pain score dropped down to 3 and he had no further need for indomethacin. Indeed, he was so delighted with his newfound comfort that he declined further measures that might have managed the residual pain. The spironolactone probably had still more effect with increasing time.

My third case in point is Evelyn D #40. Evelyn came to see me at age 81. Diagnosed earlier with gouty arthritis, she had been told by her previous doctor that the cartilage in her knees was severely damaged, and that replacement surgery would be necessary for the right knee. Meanwhile she was given periodic cortisone injections to ease the pain.

Through the usual method we established Evelyn's baseline total pain score to be 24. I brought it down to 5 with a prednisone induction. The FED dropped the score down to zero as she removed the reactive coffee and beef from her diet. These days she only occasionally uses Microdose prednisone. Evelyn's right knee, the one slated for surgical replacement, usually has no pain at all and functions entirely normally.

Evelyn thus joins many other rheumatic patients in my practice who have been able to cancel joint replacement surgery because they no longer needed it. See EC #11 in Chapter 4 and CZ #36 in Chapter 8, whose joints also healed rapidly, apparently completely, as soon as the offending antigen was removed. Evelyn's recovery demonstrates that even in the situation of eroded cartilage and where bone is reportedly rubbing on bone, there can still be satisfactory healing if the underlying inflammatory process can be halted completely. I cannot attest to whether the synovia and cartilage return to precisely the condition they were in before the gouty arthritis occurred, but it really doesn't matter, since our main objective is normal comfort and normal function.

I judge that glucosamine, after the etiologic antigen has been removed, may be of auxiliary value in healing of cartilage surfaces. Patient AA #27 in Chapter 7 might have obtained the last measure of comfort for her knees from additional use of glucosamine sulfate. Glucosamine may also enhance the health of collagen of the skin and esophagus which are attacked in scleroderma.

My 72-year-old patient, Andy C #41, had been on allopurinol maintenance for seven years. His gouty arthritis total pain score of 27 was reduced to 6 by alternate-day B12 shots.

Back in 1952, Harrington reported that red blood cells in pernicious anemia had an elevated uric acid content. This suggests to me that B12 may have a beneficial connection with the cellular metabolism of uric acid. At this time I am unable to determine whether the B12 enhanced uric acid metabolism, improved phagocytosis of immune complexes or increased hypothalamic production of CRF. Andy's improvement verifies that gouty arthritis acts at least partly like a rheumatic disease.

The fact that only 30 percent of people with an elevated blood uric acid develop gouty arthritis and that 10 percent of those with a true gouty arthritis have a normal blood uric acid, rather clearly suggests that the blood level of uric acid is not at all critical for the existence of active gout. It further suggests that the crystal formation within the joint is not reliant upon the intensity of the uric acid supply from the circulating blood. I propose that the joint crystal formation is primarily dependent upon the abnormal uric acid metabolism occurring within the joint itself.

Scientists have determined that a blood uric acid of 6.8 or greater represents full saturation and should theoretically crystallize out, thereby forming the painful crystal deposits associated with gout. But many people with much higher levels of blood uric acid have no such crystals and people with much smaller concentrations experience "impossible crystallization" in their joints, as was the situation with Julie L #38.

It is my belief that the crystals are precipitated locally in the joints in response to inherited abnormalities in local tissue metabolism, and further, that these abnormalities can lead to the local production of uric acid crystals or calcium crystals, or even both crystals, in the same person and in the same joint. The abnormal, concentrated local production of either uric acid or calcium leads to local crystallization in the joint before diffusion into the blood can occur. The only influence that an elevated circulating blood level may have upon joint crystals would be to slow down the normal diffusion of these chemicals from their joint formation site into the circulating blood for excretion by the kidneys.

The presence of joint crystals during a flare-up of gouty arthritis can be demonstrated by aspiration of the affected joint with a needle. Yet even after inflammation has ceased and healing has taken place, a follow-up aspiration of the joint will reveal the same crystals still in residence, this time without pain or swelling. This strange finding gives us a clue that the pain and inflammation of gouty arthritis must be caused, or at least initiated, by some basic irritative-inflammatory process other than the crystals. You have already learned that the crystals are coated with apoprotein during quiescence, and I believe they become recoated with the gamma globulins of immune complexes to make them more attractive to phaging by the white cells. It is the immune complexes which initiate the acute inflammation in the joint. I believe that if no crystals were present, the episode of inflammation would occur anyway, but perhaps with a lesser intensity.

The fact that the same uric acid crystals have occasionally been found in other forms of arthritis, such as rheumatoid arthritis, lupus, osteoarthritis and psoriatic arthritis, also makes their essential, etiologic role in gout less believable. The relationship between rheumatic arthritis and gout is underscored by my successful treatment of gout by methods that do not manipulate uric acid levels or crystals, but do manipulate immune complexes.

Another factor of possible significance in unraveling the gout mystery is that gout doesn't usually show up until a candidate reaches age 40 or later. It could be coincidence, but that is the age at which standard rheumatic diseases start appearing more frequently, because of an increasing production of immune complexes and because of a decreasing ability of the body's defensive systems to deal with the complexes and the inflammation they trigger.

Add to this the statistic that, although elevated blood uric acid levels occur almost routinely in kidney disease failure, less than one percent of these patients develop gout. And hundreds of thousands of women exhibit high blood uric acids in toxemia of pregnancy, yet there seem to be no reported cases of toxemia-associated gouty arthritis at all.

Precipitating Factors for Active Gout

Based on all the preceding evidence, I have developed a radically different theory of gout's origins: that *excess immune complexes* produce the primary joint irritation-inflammation. The crystals are a response to that immune irritation rather than its cause. If crystals were primary for irritation, then irritation would never stop, because crystals are always there, regardless of irritation activity. When circumstances conclude the supply of joint-irritating immune complexes, the joint will cool off, globulins will be replaced by apoproteins—a cyclicity not dissimilar to palindromic arthritis with a definite start and an end.

It should be noted that you do not necessarily have pain when immune complexes are in action. The immune complexes can work silently with irritation, as they do in osteoarthritis with silent bone deformation, and silently in the kidney as they slowly injure the kidney to reduce its filtering capabilities. Calcium crystals are very common associates in the silent joints of osteoarthritis. I suspect that in the early years of gout the small number of excess complexes only make irritation that can make crystals which will be in place at a later time when the big inflammations arise with huge numbers of immune complexes. This silent immune irritation is my explanation for crystals being present in joints of people who have never had any apparent gouty arthritis, or in joints never inflamed in people with active, painful gouty arthritis. The pattern of joints to be involved is set genetically.

One might argue that the silent irritation is a peculiar response among a select group of people who are just not reactive to the crystals, and the white cells don't attempt to eat them up. But if we then consider patients with acute gout in one joint and totally asymptomatic crystals in other joints, we are forced to conclude that such an argument is invalid.

I believe that the joint tissues of gout are in relatively poor health because of double trouble: first, because they have abnormal uric acid metabolism to make them weaker and more susceptible to inflammation; and, second, because they are cursed with immune complex irritation/ inflammation reactivity. This explains why allopurinol, even while it functions effectively in controlling the production of uric acid, is only partially successful in reducing pain (of immune complexes).

NODULES UNDER THE SKIN—TOPHI

In this section I would like to show you how very much alike gout and rheumatic diseases are in their inflammatory nodules. I believe that the cellular reaction and swelling of a tophus is induced by immune complex reactivity and that the crystal formation is secondary to and produced by the inflammatory cells of that tophus.

Microscopic examination of nodules of rheumatoid arthritis reveals some central dead tissue surrounded by cells typical of chronic immune irritation, and scar tissue. The nodules of gouty tophi also contain central dead debris surrounded by a ring of immune inflammation cells and some scar tissue. Typical of tophi, the uric acid crystals, though absent at first, form in the centers of the rings. The crystals become more numerous, and small centers unite to become large centers. This anatomical arrangement suggests that the inflammation cells contribute to the manufacture and concentration of the uric acid crystal formation in the centers which have no circulation. The highly concentrated, locally produced liquid uric acid, which has no circulation to dilute it, may crystallize in the tophus's center. It is reasonable to assume that the same type of immune complexes which form rheumatic nodules also form gouty tophi, particularly since crystals have also been found in nodules of patients with lupus and rheumatoid arthritis.

Since the dead, debris-filled centers of these tophi are surrounded by immune, phagocytic-type cells at first, and then crystals start appearing in the centers later, it seems clear to me that the particular manufacturers of uric acid for the crystals are the congregated immune cells. Tiny microtophi appear in the membranes which form the joint lining in great numbers. They form crystals, and instead of forming a large tophus, they rupture into the joint space to discharge their crystals. As long as there is immune irritation, crystals will keep forming and crystals will be constantly dissolving and then carried away as they diffuse into the circulation. I propose that there must be immune irritation for crystals to be present, and that makes the basic etiology of gout an excess immune complex disease, as with other types of arthritis. The immune complex activity also silently attacks the kidneys to slowly diminish their ability to excrete uric acid.

Up to 30 percent of tophaceous gout patients also have a positive rheumatoid arthritis factor and 7.5 percent of RA patients have an elevated uric acid.

Kidneys and Immune Complexes

My research also leads me to believe that the crystals that form within the kidney tissues are also produced in response to immune complex irritation of the kidneys. This is because the irritation is slow to develop and mild in its initial manifestations, not the furious commotion that may occur in the joint inflammations. The resulting irritation and kidney damage results not only in increasingly high blood uric acid, but also in hypertension, which occurs in about 44 percent of patients with established diagnoses of gout. This expands the concept of kidney involvement, since the hypertension could arise from irritation of the juxtaglomerular apparatus, which is a link in the chain of hypertension. Similar kidney irritations contribute to the increased uric acid found in many lupus and RA patients. In the past, when gout was not treated with our modern medicines, a goodly number of gout patients died as the result of kidney failure.

A Radical Approach to Treatment

I have used "unorthodox" measures to treat my gout patients with beneficial results that are far in excess of those of standard therapy. I use the term unorthodox here to describe my use of immune complex reduction therapy, and I can say conservatively that I have achieved improvements over my patients' previous treatments ranging from 30 percent at the low end to 97 percent in some cases.

My successful therapy for gouty arthritis has three main objectives. First, to reduce the number of immune complexes produced, as in my other arthritis therapies, by removing or blocking antigens. Second, to strengthen the body's natural anti-inflammatory defenses with vitamin and prednisone supplementation. And third, to reduce the intensity of the abnormal uric acid cellular metabolism with both allopurinol and spironolactone.

Though medical reports incriminate diuretics, notably the thiazides, in the precipitation of gouty arthritis, yet my primary therapeutic agent in the treatment of gout is the diuretic spironolactone. Diuretics reduce the volume of water in the body by increasing the amount of water passed in the urine. As the volume of circulating blood is also reduced, diuretics are often thought to be directly responsible for raising the blood uric acid concentrations; but that elevation, on the contrary, results mostly from the reduced renal excretion of uric acid by the thiazide inhibition. I find spironolactone to have certain unique capabilities that make it nonetheless well suited to gout therapy. Chiefly, spironolactone reduces abnormal uric acid metabolism about 20 percent, while it also decreases kidney excretion of uric acid about 20 percent, so there is no change in the blood levels of uric acid. The profit is not in a better, measurable blood test, but in healthier cells. At the same time, spironolactone may effectively reduce the activity of hormonal antigen for double-barreled protection in gouty arthritis.

For safety, be sure to have your potassium and creatinine levels checked before using spironolactone (see Chapter 7), but if indications are favorable, use it with confidence. Note that my therapy does not include colchicine, one of the more widely used pain relievers for treating acute gout. Colchicine works by inhibiting phagocytosis and the resultant production of inflammatory chemicals, and thereby depresses the immune system. My therapeutic approach to all rheumatic disease is to *enhance* the immune system. The use of colchicine has ceased in some countries, such as England, because it is believed to have more dangers than other more conservative measures.

When the diagnosis of acute gout has been verified and the laboratory values of blood potassium and creatinine have been determined to be normal, I immediately start a program of daily spironolactone 100 mg and allopurinol 200 mg along with injected B12 1,000 mcg and oral megavitamins as previously outlined in Chapter 5. Prednisone is given 10-10-5-5-5 mg for five days. When symptoms have been thoroughly controlled, I very slowly decrease the B12 and allopurinol to lesser doses, but only as tolerated. If there are small, residual daily symptoms, the next step is to hunt for the reaction-causing antigen, using the FED first. If there are no residual symptoms, then I would use the blood uric acid level as a guide for allopurinol dosage. Weight control is also in order. It's safe to say that anyone who wants to get relief of pain and inflammation for sensitive joints ought, at very least, to work on shedding the excess pounds which add so much to mechanical stress. With the diet, diminish the purine foods such as liver, fowl, sardines and legumes, and coffee and other caffeine drinks.

Vitamin B12 could theoretically increase joint pain by enhancing phagocytosis of crystals, but in my view, its ability to enhance systemic phagocytosis of immune complexes makes a far more compelling argument in its favor. The reason is this: with excess immune complexes eliminated, the various inflammatory responses do not occur, and the attack of gout can thereby be inhibited.

For readers with a technical bent, here are some other interesting details giving a favorable view of B12 that I would like to share with you. Harrigan in 1952 reported that the red blood cells in pernicious anemia had an elevated uric acid content, while the red cells after B12 therapy had a normal content. B12 is involved in converting dihydrofolic acid into tetrahydrofolic acid, and the latter is involved in purine metabolism, which can be the source of uric acid. This suggests to me that B12 may have a beneficial connection with the cellular metabolism of uric acid. The biochemist Styer writes in 1995 that the biochemical lesion in most cases of gout has not been elucidated, and that a small portion of gout patients have abnormal xanthine metabolism to make excess uric acid. That leaves the basic abnormality open to some conjecture.

LIFETIME OF GOUT

Research indicates that persons who develop gout in later life actually arrive on Earth with a predisposition to the disease. In other words, they are born with genetically altered metabolic function but have not had the time to develop immune sensitivities. Further, their increased uric acid production goes unnoticed in blood tests, because all the excess is easily excreted by normally functioning kidneys.

At the time of puberty a whole new set of hormones comes into play, to which immune sensitivity frequently develops. At about age 20 immune irritation may start diminishing kidney function so that some people are starting on the road to an elevated blood level of uric acid. During the asymptomatic years, immune joint irritation may start the silent deposition of crystals from increased tissue uric acid production, mostly by white mononuclear cells.

Between the ages of 30 and 40 a few males will start with symptomatic gouty arthritis acute inflammation, which is superimposed upon joints previously only silently irritated. After age 40 many more males and some females show active inflammatory disease. Starting around the fiftieth year, the symptoms of gouty arthritis become more persistent from day to day. Visible tophi may start forming in their usual locations. When the blood uric acid levels rise as a result of kidney immune irritation, it becomes more likely, but not certain, that there will be more active gouty arthritis disease. The time of kidney irritation also brings nearly a 50 percent incidence of hypertension. If the condition is neglected, the consequences to the joint and kidney can be severe; but, if it is treated carefully, the future should be comfortable and without serious damage.

Virtually all medical authorities are agreed on the genetic factor for abnormal uric acid metabolism as a fundamental in gouty arthritis. Not yet recognized is the fact that the individual must also inherit a predisposition to produce an excess of immune complexes specific to triggering the irritated/inflammatory joint and kidney disease patterns of gouty arthritis. There is probably a linked inheritance of the above factors, because they are so frequently expressed together in a unique pattern of joint and kidney disease.

Gout is predominantly a disease of joint membranes and cartilage, with microtophi occurring in abundance in the synovia. I suspect that glucosamine might have a favorable effect at this location if discomforts cannot be chased away by antigen removal.

REMEMBER

1. Gout is a heritable disease involving abnormalities in the body's uric acid metabolism and in the immune system's production of excess immune complexes. The kidneys are almost always the target of immune irritation, as well as the painful joints.
2. Local accumulations of uric acid crystals may occur in joints as a metabolic response to immune irritation.
3. Immune complex irritability is primarily responsible for active

gouty arthritis, for kidney irritation, and for crystal formation in the joint tissues and tophi.

4. Crystals may be inactive when coated with apoprotein and become phagocytically reactive when coated with immunoglobulins supplied by immune complexes.

5. The drug allopurinol markedly decreases abnormal uric acid metabolism to improve cellular health, to improve pain symptoms and to lower blood uric acid.

6. Spironolactone, either alone or in synergistic combination with allopurinol, is a very effective and safe method for preventing acute gout and controlling chronic gouty arthritis.

7. Gouty arthritis may be controlled by other measures that reduce immune complexes and/or control inflammation, such as the FED, antibiotic therapy, prednisone and appropriate megavitamins.

8. Eroded joint surfaces may heal if the irritant antigens are completely removed.

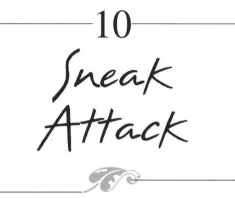

10
Sneak Attack

INFECTIOUS AGENTS AS A SOMETIME
FACTOR IN ARTHRITIS

W<small>E HAVE</small> already learned that both foods and hormones can play a role in arthritis through their formation of immune complexes. Now we will focus on the part that infectious agents play in the same disease of arthritis.

Since the beginning of rheumatology, considerable attention has been paid to bacteria and viruses and their possible roles in initiating and perpetuating rheumatic disease. This information has been so elusive and the opinions so varied that the real truth has slipped through our scientific fingers. Still, no one can ignore the fact that some patients experience an abrupt onset of rheumatic disease in a manner that seems to insist on infection having been involved.

Part of the reason for so much uncertainty in the past is that arthritis turns out to be the result of a number of quite different factors that produce just one and the same disease. This problem is similar to cancer, which has many causes but also many expressions. We now know that microbial infections are indeed a trigger for arthritis, and that as infectious agents they are antigenic, capable of triggering an immune antibody response in the body. But bacteria are just one of the three groups of antigenic factors.

The arthritis disease experienced is not directly the result of the germ itself, but rather the body's reaction to the immune chemicals generated by that organism. To cite just one example of how complicated the chain of cause and effect can be, I will mention a study some years ago, by Szanto et al. (1983) of a group of women who were uniformly diagnosed with severe pelvic infection. Rheumatic low back pain, called sacroiliitis, developed among some of them, but only in those whose inherited tissue type was known as HLA-B27. Those without that inherited factor developed no arthritis at all.

Much of what we do know about the causal relationship between infections and arthritis comes from fifty years of investigation by Thomas McPherson Brown, M.D. In his enjoyably-written autobiography, *The Road Back*, he describes his career-long effort to develop his theory of cause and effect, and the tetracycline therapy that grew out of it. A cornerstone of his discoveries was his development of a technique for culturing fluids withdrawn from rheumatic joints to demonstrate the not-infrequent presence of mycoplasma. Mycoplasmas are a unique group of organisms that share characteristics of both bacteria and viruses. Though they are as small as viruses and, like them, have no cell walls, they are capable of living and reproducing outside living cells, making them remarkably viable infectious agents. One reason that mycoplasma was often not isolated by culture from a joint was simply that it was not there—the mycoplasma was growing elsewhere or the arthritis was caused by another antigenic factor. The presence of obscure mycoplasma anywhere in the body can now be detected by testing for specific antibodies to them in the blood and also by improved techniques for culture, but there is no question in my mind that Dr. Brown led the way.

Mycoplasmas live mostly on the surface of mucous membranes along the respiratory and the urogenital tracts, and their antigens are absorbed through the membranes. About 50 percent or more of the general human population tests positive for mycoplasmas, which more often than not produce no symptoms. When symptoms do appear, they can usually be routed by tetracycline or other related antibiotics.

However, there are times when the mycoplasma may invade the human host and be transported by the blood to distant tissues and organs. The circumstances favoring such an invasion are related to a depression of immune resistance. Those patients who take immuno-suppressive drugs as part of cancer chemotherapy, or in conjunction with organ transplantation, have an increased susceptibility to myco-plasma infection.

We know that patients immunocompromised by normal preg-nancy have mycoplasma as the cause of at last half of their postpar-tum infections and fevers, and their low birth weight deliveries are associated with an increased mycoplasma infection of the fetal mem-branes and uterus. Profoundly immunodepressed AIDS patients have a high incidence of invasive mycoplasma infections too.

Because mycoplasma organisms can trigger responses in remote sites either by invasion themselves or by sending immune complex spinoffs, it can be very difficult to gather clear proof of their type of involvement in cases of arthritis. Good diagnostic capabilities are restricted to a few research centers. An antibody technique for de-tecting mycoplasma is widely available, but positive findings prove only the presence of mycoplasma, not specifically where it is. Fortu-nately, however, other than for scientific understanding, it really doesn't matter much where the inflammation originates, because tak-ing the proper antibiotic should eliminate the immune reactions as well as the infections, wherever they may be.

Spread of mycoplasma from one person to another may occur upon very close contact with the respiratory or genital system of an infected person. If only one spouse is treated and cleared of all mycoplasma, it is likely that there will soon be a reinfection from the mate, so antibiotic therapy is generally in order for both of them. About 25 percent of infants are colonized with mycoplasma at birth. For just a few of them, the incubation time is three weeks, and then an illness may last for a month or so before subsiding. This could be a source of juvenile rheumatoid arthritis.

Even though mycoplasma is not producing any symptoms of direct irritation, your body may be host to some antigen-antibody activity which your natural defenses are able to absorb and neutralize silently. Then one day, possibly in later years, something disturbs the balance of control. You may have a severe injury or break a bone. You may get a severe infection or you may have a great emotional upset. You may eat an excessive amount of food to which you have become reactive. Or it may be simply that the mycoplasmas have multiplied to the extent that their complexes alone are overwhelming you. Whatever it may be, you are now at risk of inflammation because your defensive systems are being overtaxed. Injuries may appear to heal but their residual inflammatory pains remain. Pains may sometimes arise for no apparent reason and then just go away . . . or *not* go away!

Ordinary bacteria at times may also produce arthritis. Chronic streptococcal infection is one condition in which it has been recognized that they are the culprits. When recognized, the infection is usually brought under control with a regimen of penicillin.

A relatively new and increasing source of infection-triggered arthritis is Lyme disease, which is caused by the bite of a deer tick infected with the bacterium *Borrelia burgdorferi*. Identification of the onset of Lyme disease can often be made through examination of the type of tick, by some rather typical rashes, and by blood testing. A short course of antibiotics may take care of Lyme if diagnosed early. But if the infection goes unnoticed and is allowed to progress to joint inflammation, usually several weeks after the infection has had a chance to become systemic, full recovery can be difficult and uncertain.

People whose tissues are of the HLA-B27 type are usually susceptible to a variety of infections associated with immune complex production, the women with associated infection and low back pain cited earlier being a good example. A disease called Reiter's syndrome or reactive arthritis is another manifestation. Reiter's syndrome usually develops after an individual contracts nonspecific urethritis or dysentery, and may be the result of any one of several infectious agents, some strange, some familiar, including salmonella, yersinia, chlamydia, ureaplasma and HIV. As the infection spreads, it may induce added symptoms of conjunctivitis, mouth sores and arthritis, the latter commonly in the knees or ankle. Tendons and ligaments may also become tender and inflamed, and the whole complex may linger for periods of a few days to several months. At times, the arthritis may become chronic from continued infestation by the microbe.

Rheumatic bacterial infections, like mycoplasma infections, can cause inflammation far from the site of the invasion. In contrast to the behavior of bacteria entering a cut in the skin and causing local redness, swelling, heat and pain from the direct effect of toxins, the bacteria of rheumatic disease may produce no signs of where they are growing locally; rather, the resulting inflammation is found in distant joints as an indirect response to immune complexes arising from the bacteria's antigenic factors.

ANTIBIOTIC THERAPY FOR ARTHRITIS

The mycoplasma agent in arthritis was found by Dr. Brown, who experimented at length with antibiotics in treating arthritis-mycoplasma problems. He found them to be responsive to just small amounts of tetracycline administered only three days a week. I do not personally have extensive first-hand experience in the use of tetracycline therapy, because it is still relatively new as a concept. But I have long been aware of microbes as one of the three potential sources of antigen, because logic told me it would have to be. The information from Dr. Brown's book and The Road Back Foundation expands upon that aspect and fits well into my preconceived pattern.

Remarkably, when the antibiotic is first administered, there is sometimes, but not always, a distinct increase of rheumatic symptoms, and often some new ones as well. This is the so-called Jarisch-Herxheimer reaction, which includes pain, dizziness and sometimes loose bowel movements and is due to the rapid release of the dying mycoplasma's toxic contents. The reaction may continue for a week or so. If it should happen to you, try to find the positive in it: it means that the battle is joined and you will ultimately get significant relief from your disease. With my own patients, I do my best to lower the risk of Herxheimer reaction by introducing the tetracycline slowly, starting at 250 mg three times a week and then building to 750 or 1,000 mg thrice weekly. The speed at which I make the increases and the size of the maximum doses is governed by how the patient reacts. After one to four months the total pain score should begin to diminish, and then, with good luck, it will slowly descend to near zero.

Dr. Brown theorized that the longer the disease had been instituted in body tissues, the more fortified the entrenched mycoplasmas become, and therefore the longer the therapy required to dislodge them. Though some experts disagree on this point, Dr. Brown's basic therapeutic concepts have been determined to be correct by N.I.H. studies, and perhaps the tissue invasiveness concept will also be proven correct with time.

Tetracycline therapy may be extended from a minimum of four months to possibly as long as two years or even more. The decline of symptoms to zero or a prolonged plateau will suggest when the therapy is complete, though blood tests comparing antibodies before and after therapy can be used as additional evidence. I assume from Dr. Brown's statements that up to 80 percent of his patients experienced an average of 80 percent symptom relief from this method of therapy. Regrettably, Dr. Brown did not have an equivalent of my Daily Total Pain Score by which to make more specific evaluations and reports.

I have been using the term tetracycline loosely to refer not only to the original tetracycline, but also to the other members of the tetracycline drug family, including doxycycline and minocycline, or Minocin. Minocycline is a relatively new member of the tetracycline family, milder in effect and more commonly used to treat acne. It reputedly has a more penetrating effect on certain mycoplasmas and is less likely to promote yeast infections or increase sensitivity to sunlight, two unfortunate side effects of antibiotic therapy. However, it can cause dizziness and it should not be taken with iron supplements, which inactivate it. The dosage varies from 50 to 200 mg three times a week, or even daily for severe cases. The current price of minocycline is about 44 times greater than tetracycline, or about $90 instead of $2 per month. When the rare resistance to any of the tetracyclines occurs, erythromycin or clindamycin can be substituted with favorable results.

Because patients with rheumatic disease are generally immuno-compromised to some degree, I like to enhance antibiotic control of the disease with large doses of vitamins E, C, B1 and beta-carotene and B12 injections; together, these supplements increase both anti-body production and the destruction of bacteria by phagocytosis.

WHEN TO CONCLUDE ANTIBIOTIC THERAPY

Many people harbor the mycoplasma germs for years and never have a single rheumatic symptom. Then, one day, symptoms arrive. How come? Once again, I find this occurrence a confirmation of my theory that rheumatic disease is caused when the number of immune complexes in the body exceeds the ability of the defensive systems to counteract and destroy them. In this additive process, immune complexes from foods, hormones and bacteria may all play a part. If the rate of immune complex production from mycoplasmas exceeds the body's defensive threshold, then rheumatic symptoms will be produced by the mycoplasma alone; if not, the patient will be asymptomatic until something else occurs to overwhelm the defenses and acute disease blossoms.

To see how this might work, we will suppose that an individual with subliminal mycoplasma infection starts taking the female hormone progestin in the form of menopausal hormones. The progestin pill may introduce a small amount of immune complexes, which might ordinarily cause no symptomatic reaction. But in this case, the progestin complexes are being created in a body already sustaining a borderline quantity of mycobacterial immune complexes. The combination of these two might well rise above the defensive threshold and result in rheumatic inflammation. If at this point one were either to eliminate the mycoplasma infection by tetracycline, or to halt the action of progestin by stopping the progestin medication, the result would be exactly the same—reduction of total immune complexes and therefore pain relief. Alternatively, the patient might get similar pain relief as the result of megadosage vitamin therapy that boosts the activity of the defensive systems.

The ideal end point of medical therapy is usually considered to be zero symptoms. However, one must look upon antibiotic rheumatic therapy somewhat differently. More important than getting rid of all the symptoms is the complete elimination of all microbes from the body, for if they are not *all* eliminated, there is always the potential for their regrowth. Criteria for having accomplished complete removal of mycoplasma could be a finding of zero mycoplasma antibody in the blood, or establishment of a zero total pain score.

A finding of zero antibodies in the blood is not a totally reliable test. Its unreliability is reflected in the fact that some physicians routinely treat rheumatoid arthritis antibiotically, even in the absence of a positive blood test, on the grounds that the antibody factors may not always be detected with current diagnostic techniques. Presumably a more reliable detection system will be developed in the future.

A zero pain score is also not always a workable criterion. When we have reduced the mycoplasma population to below the rheumatic disease threshold and there are zero pain symptoms, it does not mean that the mycoplasma has necessarily been eliminated from the body, because a subliminal infection could still be brewing.

Another problem with relying solely upon the pain score arises when there is also a reactive food that can independently exceed the pain threshold. In this circumstance, although the mycoplasma may have been totally removed by the antibiotic, the symptoms, although certainly diminished, will still be present because of the food. In the first proposition, the mycoplasma was incompletely treated in spite of zero symptoms, while in the second proposition, the mycoplasma was totally eliminated by the antibiotic in spite of the persistence of pain. The problem is how to manage therapy so that there is neither excessive nor inadequate utilization of the antibiotic.

For the purpose of establishing a more reliable, realistic, zero-pain score objective, I would first go through the much shorter-term and relatively simpler therapies designed to eliminate or control antigen factors arising from diet or hormones. The defensive systems should also be beefed up to maximum performance. If symptoms still remain, it now becomes practicable to initiate a course of antibiotic therapy for however long it takes to control microbial rheumatic disease with the ultimate aim of achieving zero pain.

When the point of zero pain has been reached, I generally continue antibiotic therapy for an additional time to eliminate any residual, undetectable mycoplasma. My practice is to continue four months beyond the cessation of pain. Those cases that take longer to control suggest that there is a slower response of the mycoplasma, and accordingly would profit from a longer total therapy.

Let us consider a theoretical rheumatic patient whose baseline total pain score is 100. Through the FED, coffee is identified as the troublemaker, and the score comes down to 75. Then I add estrogen and progestin and further reduce the score to 50. Next, I add spironolactone, lowering the score to 25. Finally, I put the patient on antibiotic therapy, and over the course of six months the score slowly descends to zero. At this point I have the patient continue the antibiotic for another four months as a sort of insurance policy against regrowth. Though the future can never be guaranteed, the patient can be said to be "cured" for the present. I want to note that attaining a zero pain score does not mean the end of immune complexes, because they must be formed daily as part of survival against the invading bacterial world, but the end of *excessive* immune complexes!

There is no doubt in my mind about the potential effectiveness of tetracyclines, and a report from a large multicenter study by the N.I.H. confirms that it is safe and effective. Recent reports from Israel and other medical centers suggest that about half of the treated patients experience improvement, with an average 50 percent reduction in pain and other symptoms. The longer the patients were on the antibiotics, the greater the improvement. A few patients stopped their antibiotic when in disease remission, but soon found the necessity for resuming medication because of returning symptoms. This perhaps represents either a regrowth of mycoplasma or reinfection from a mate.

Based on these findings and the fact that I have obtained about 70 percent overall pain relief for my patients in the past without having used tetracycline therapy as an adjunct, I am confident that patients treated with the combination of therapies, including tetracycline therapy, can look forward to as much as 90 percent average relief.

I have one interesting patient to report for whom tetracycline therapy produced some good and unpredicted results. I took on Joseph I #42 as a patient at the age of 62 in 1984. Joe described to me the gradual onset of osteoarthritis over some 20 years. At the age of 61 he experienced a huge surge of inflammation and pain in his low back, chest, neck, hips, knees, abdomen, right wrist and hand. He also had edema of the entire right leg and thigh. A blood test taken by a rheumatologist he had been seeing tested positive for antinuclear antibodies. X-rays showed osteoarthritic changes of the right knee. NSAIDs had effected little to no relief of pain and his condition worsened when he contracted a series of staphylococcal infections.

It was shortly after that Joe agreed to try my unconventional therapy. After we established a baseline total pain score of 60, I began medicating Joe with Provera 10 mg daily. He experienced better relief of pain than with the NSAIDs, but still was very much in pain. I then switched him to spironolactone 100 mg daily. This proved highly effective in reducing pain and swelling within a few days, and over the next two months his total pain score tumbled down to 4. Meanwhile, Joe determined that he had adverse pain reactions to caffeine and coffee, so he eliminated them from his diet.

Some time later, in 1992, Joe's arthritis flared up again when he was involved in an auto accident, and the total pain score rose up to 12 and remained at that level. When Joe reported in with his latest arthritis flare-up, I prescribed Microdose prednisone. As the pain subsided, dropping in a short time to 2, we found Joe could go as long as six months between Microdosing.

However, in 1993 Joe reported that during the previous two years he noticed an increasingly irregular heartbeat, which was accompanied in the last few months by shortness of breath after even mild exertion. There was a slight increase of joint discomfort, for a pain score of 5. Also, during the previous year, Joe had developed a sensitivity to black pepper which produced rather severe pains of the lower abdomen, pelvis and thighs. When Joe eliminated the pepper, he eliminated that problem.

With the possibility of an underlying infection in mind, I tested Joe's mycoplasma titer and found it was low positive. Accordingly, I put him on increasing doses of tetracycline three times a week. Within two weeks of starting the antibiotic, Joe began to notice slight improvements, and by six weeks he could scarcely measure his joint pain or muscle stiffness. Surprisingly, Joe's heart was showing signs of recovery; his heart rhythm returned to normal rhythm at rest, and his shortness of breath was diminishing. Even more surprising, Joe's sensitivity to pepper disappeared. After 18 months of tetracycline therapy Joe could do eight hours of heavy physical labor with no pains or heart problems. To put it simply, someone who acted like an old person had been reborn as a relative youngster.

I had expected the tetracycline therapy to help Joe's mild arthritis, which it did, but Joe's improved heart was a special bonus. My best explanation is that Joe had a mycoplasma-induced immune complex heart muscle inflammation, or myocarditis. It is unlikely that the mycoplasma infection was localized in the heart, as mycoplasmas usually colonize only the surface membranes of the respiratory and genital tracts.

As for Joe's sensitivity to pepper disappearing with tetracycline therapy, I remain puzzled. When the tetracycline was discontinued for three weeks, the pepper sensitivity returned strongly; when medication was resumed, it went away. I wish I had the answer for all events in life!

Tetracycline has been tested in and recommended for rheumatoid arthritis, but another form of arthritis involving the skin, called scleroderma, has also been reported to respond well. It is generally believed that the treatment of osteoarthritis with tetracycline would be of no avail, but Joe's experience shows otherwise. The critical point is that for the antibiotic to work, there must be mycoplasma infection present in the first place; but since it is often difficult to determine its presence for certain, I am not averse to the idea of trying tetracycline even in the absence of clear evidence for infection if more obvious therapies don't work. As stated before, I proceed on the basis that all antigen-managing therapies are applicable to all forms of arthritis regardless of what name might be attached to them.

We are living at a time when investigations into a bacterium called chlamydia may reveal to us new sources of immune disease. Chlamydia, like mycoplasma, is a common inhabitant of our bodies, only chlamydia must live within our cells rather than on the surface. They both may inhabit the same body and they both respond to the same antibiotics.

DOES TETRACYCLINE PROTECT BONE-JOINT INTEGRITY?

As with all tissues of our bodies, our normal bones and cartilage are constantly being removed and replaced. When bone is removed more than replaced, as in osteoporosis, a problem disease state is produced by the deficit. Cartilage dissolution for removal is done by zinc metalloproteinases, such as collagenase and gelatinase. As collagenase destroys cartilage, a chemical called pyridinoline is formed and excreted through the urine. In rheumatic and osteoarthritis there are increased amounts of pyridinoline in the urine. Scientists have observed that tetracycline may reduce the urinary pyridinoline, reduce joint free oxygen radicals, inhibit proteolytic enzymes, stimulate cartilage growth and inhibit the aging of cartilage cells, called chondrocytes.

I think it is debatable whether tetracycline actually has all these good, *direct* biochemical effects. I favor the concept that the improved joint health status arises *indirectly* from the reduced joint immune complex reactivity (irritation/inflammation) which follows the killing of the mycoplasma. I have found that removal of any of the food, hormonal or bacterial antigens may result in the rapid and complete healing of severely involved joints —with or without the use of tetracycline or glucosamine.

Dr. Brown's tetracycline-mycoplasma-arthritis theories were sufficiently radical to have been met with resistance for fifty years from the medical community—to the end of his life. Shortly after Dr. Brown died, his ideas were officially tested, and now they are recognized as being very important.

REMEMBER

1. Mycoplasma is a unique group of microorganisms with characteristics of both viruses and bacteria.
2. Mycoplasma infections may last a lifetime.
3. Mycoplasma makes the continuing production of antigen to make immune complexes.
4. There are no rheumatic symptoms until the production of immune complexes quantitatively exceeds the neutralizing capability of the defensive systems.
5. Tetracycline in small doses kills mycoplasma.
6. To be maximally effective, tetracycline therapy should be followed for extended periods, ranging from four months to several years.
7. As there is no completely reliable test to determine who really harbors the mycoplasma, therapy must often be undertaken on a trial and error basis.

11

Management of Painless Osteoarthritis

A VANITY AFFAIR

THE SILENT bony alterations of osteoarthritis have been exceedingly difficult to manage. Osteoarthritis is very commonly associated with pain and occasionally with swelling. It is logical to consider that the pain, swelling and bone changes, which may occur simultaneously, are all due to only one disease process, and that would be of immune complex reactivity. That reactivity may consist of inflammation, which is represented by redness, swelling, pain and tenderness, or of irritation, which is altered cellular function, and which is represented by weakness, stiffness, paralysis, numbness, anesthesia and altered bone growth.

Many people experience virtually painless distortion of their finger joints. The altered bone growth is a very slow process with only imperceptible changes occurring within an observation period of a day, week or month. If an exactly correct therapeutic measure were to be undertaken, it could not be confirmed by even exacting bone observations until after six months or a year. Without the guiding element of pain, our measurement of success becomes almost impracticably slow and thereby makes the finding of a successful therapeutic measure very difficult, slow and inevitably inexact.

It may be exceedingly important to some particular people, whose fingers are threatening or have a strong potential for going out of shape, to retain their finger beauty and function either for personal ideals or for occupational excellence. A beautician may feel that unattractive hands will be detrimental to her business. A surgeon may fear that distorted fingers will interfere with his ability to do delicate operative procedures. A housewife may dread the losing of her attractiveness to her husband, or she might just want to protect her own self-image. Since these perceived threats of the future cannot be verified until the future arrives, nothing can ordinarily be done about it until it is already too late and the distortions have become irrevocably established. One way of looking into the future is to look at the fingers of your mother and father, which you are likely, but not certain, to duplicate. At the present time, medical science has nothing to offer these unfortunate people other than condolences, whether they are at the inception of the problem or at the end of the line, with extensive joint disfigurement.

Rheumatic pain is the usual motivation for obtaining medical care, but beauty and function are also a most reasonable and legitimate request. Certainly countless millions of dollars are spent each year on procedures such as face lifts, breast alterations and liposuction, and those procedures carry a potential of infection or even death. It is the patient, not the doctor, who should make the primary decision whether it is reasonable or not to spend the time and the money working with these simple, nontoxic arthritis medications. The risk is only to your time and your money, not your health. These medicines present essentially no danger to your health, and you may possibly be delighted with establishing the control of your painless arthritis as well as the possible improvement in your general health. It is more than fair for you to try these reasonable measures, as long as you have not been deluded into believing that there is any element of a guarantee in any one measure or even in all of them combined. I was considered to be a scientific madman when I first used spironolactone for my osteoarthritis (never so used before by anyone); but, as a consequence, I have now enjoyed thirteen years of comfort and halted bony deformation, as evidenced by X-ray comparisons, in place of devastating pain, disability and likely joint distortion. I had no data to prove the value of spironolactone before I took it, and now I have no data other than related observations to prove the value of these suggested measures for your painless osteoarthritis. Accordingly, what I will be talking about is part theory and part fact rather than established medical procedure. Nothing new is ever found out unless you try!

Since your osteoarthritis is painless, it will probably be a little beginning bone deformation that tunes you in to your potential problem. By accurate measurement of your fingers with a set of finger fitting rings and with careful tabulation of the measurements in a notebook for all eighteen joints of your ten fingers, you can establish a reliable baseline. By repeating this self examination every six months, you will obtain an impartial, objective evaluation of your condition's progress. A set of finger measuring rings can be obtained from your local jeweler for less than $10 for a plastic set, less than $20 for a stainless steel set. Things that can alter the accuracy of your finger measurements are large gains or losses of weight, the temperature and the time of day. The success that you will be looking for is a cessation of the enlargement, and I estimate that your chances for success will be in excess of 50 percent. Your hopes for any bone shrinkage in all likelihood will not be met.

If you wish to pursue the elusive chance for therapeutic control of your silent osteoarthritis, here are are my ideas:

1. Use vitamin E, vitamin C, beta-carotene and EPA, which are protective of your health even without rheumatic disease. Make sure that your vitamin D intake is adequate.
2. Use melatonin 3-5 mg each night at bedtime.
3. Give up caffeine completely, and also alcohol, because they are the most common food troublemakers and tissue irritants.
4. Have a mycoplasma and ASO antibody blood study taken. If the results are positive, take a course of the appropriate antibiotic for 12 to 24 months or more. If the test is negative, there is still a

chance that you might be harboring mycoplasma, but you would then be taking the antibiotic with a little less enthusiasm.

5. For menopausal females, use the menopausal replacement hormones of estrogen and progestin, which I believe you should be using anyway for improved quality and quantity of life.

6. Use spironolactone, particularly if you are hypertensive or have gout. Check that your kidneys are in good order.

7. Vitamin B12 injections could be given by yourself once a week, particularly if there is any associated numbness or weakness.

8. Use of the FED detection system is without value in the absence of pain as an indicator. Even though skin testing is not reliable, it might supply some inexact clues as to which foods might be eliminated from your diet.

9. The power of positive thinking and tapes for hypnotherapy and meditation for mental and physical relaxation and immune enhancement cannot have a negative influence, and they could be a profitable measure for your life and health in general.

In regard to the above nine categories, I suggest that you select all those you wish to do and act upon them now. It would take several years to test each category separately and there could be progressive distortion while you are testing. Experience tells us that there is usually more than one antigenic factor involved in producing the rheumatic problem. As you treat more than one category at a time, you will become confused as to which one was the winner, but it really doesn't matter, as long as *you* win. If you are a winner, each of the categories should be continued for the extent of your life except for the antibiotics, which might be stopped after two years or so.

There is an additional therapeutic agent that might fit into your plans for silent osteoarthritis prophylaxis. For this we must again use a little untested imagination. We do not yet understand how glucosamine sulfate bestows its beneficence upon a joint, but it is reasonable to say that it protects against biochemical erosion (by NSAIDs), enhances the health of cartilage and cartilage cells, and can replace eroded cartilage with healthy new cartilage. If we can maintain the basic health of the cartilage, it seems reasonable to think that distortion of the joints might not occur. If glucosamine is successful in this endeavor, then we will conclude that it inhibits the irritational activity of immune complexes. That would not only be logical, but somewhat expected, because glucosamine clinical testing has already demonstrated some anti-inflammatory power in osteoarthritis against immune complexes in a manner we do not yet understand. Glucosamine sulfate may be tried alone, but there would be more assuredness from using it in conjunction with the above outlined measures.

REMEMBER

I believe that there is a reasonable but unproven chance for controlling silent osteoarthritis bone changes, but the process of finding out may be exceedingly slow. You will probably meet stiff physician resistance. Cosmetic surgery presents far greater dangers and much greater cost than these simple arthritis measures, yet cosmetology has now become fully accepted by the medical community.

12
Mind-Talk

IMPROVING YOUR INTERNAL DIALOGUE
TO COMBAT STRESS-INDUCED ARTHRITIS

ALTHOUGH PHYSICIANS have traditionally made a distinction between "real" diseases and those that are psychosomatic, we now recognize that there is a two-way street between the body and the mind. As time goes on, it is becoming ever more apparent that biological events can alter psychological behavior. Various food, environmental-chemical and hormone factors can lead to such conditions as premenstrual tension, depression and psychosis. Psychological states of mind also have physiological effects: fear, anger, frustration and loss of control occasionally trigger stomach ulcers, bloody diarrhea and depression of the immune system. And emotional stress can make the experience of almost any disease measurably worse.

Ancient medicine men intuitively understood the close ties between mind and body and used it in their treatments and healing rituals. Variously known as shamans, witch doctors and priests, these traditional healers used impressive song, dance, fire and sacrificial rituals, and they administered herbal medicines and advice. Though they came from widely separated parts of the world—Africa, the Americas, the islands of the far Pacific—they shared many similarities, suggesting that there must be elements of true effectiveness in such practices for so many diverse people to believe in them.

Modern science, unfortunately, has dismissed ancient medical systems and practice in its concentration on "hard" facts and statistical data. But when scientists have taken the trouble to analyze some of the shamans' old herbs, they have discovered the bases of some of our modern pharmaceuticals. We are still very slow, however, to investigate the psychological measures of ancient medicine men— such practices as the use of curses and trances, and the removing of spells. Those scientists who have personally witnessed acts of healing are reluctant to acknowledge that the medicine men have anything but good luck working for them.

I want to show you in this chapter how the dialogues between your conscious and subconscious brain are involved not only in the maintenance of your health, but also in controlling your immune disease of arthritis. You will find that the most sensitive spot is your hypothalamus, which manages not only your feelings of happiness but also the functioning of your immune system. I will demonstrate what can really go wrong and that those wrongs can really be corrected if approached with "proper" therapies, which at times may be witch doctors. Some people may think some of this is "way out," but it is a factual part of your life.

Given that the mind is inseparably inter-connected with the body, it makes sense that to treat one without considering the other is incomplete. This is essentially what holistic medicine is all about, and it has particular relevance in regard to rheumatic disease. Anyone who suffers owes it to him/herself to work on improving the internal dialogue.

To make my point clear, I'll start with a case reported in the medical literature more than twenty years ago: A 28-year-old Philippine-American woman became severely sick with symptoms of weakness, enlarged liver and enlarged lymph nodes. Upon further examination by a Western-trained physician, she was found to have the classic findings of lupus, with low thyroid as a further complication.

Treated with high doses of prednisone and thyroid medicine, she at first improved, but soon all of her problems returned, only more severely and with the additional findings of excess steroids. Another arthritis medicine was used, but still to no advantage. Fearing that she would soon become a total invalid, she decided to visit her native country one last time.

When she arrived in her home country of the Philippines, she went to see a local witch doctor. He performed a ritual healing which climaxed with the removal of a curse that had been placed upon her by a former suitor. Feeling greatly relieved, she returned to her American lupus doctor just three weeks later. He found her no longer weak, no longer moon-faced and no longer taking medication, and she told him she was free of all her former symptoms. She refused laboratory testing in compliance with the warnings of her witch doctor.

Fourteen months later she became pregnant and ultimately delivered a healthy girl. Her only problem during pregnancy was a mild anemia. Her lupus never returned.

What can possibly explain such a reversal? Are we all capable of receiving such miraculous cures? Probably not. For curses and voodoos to be effective, the patient must be a strong believer and raised in an environment in which religious beliefs and rites are a fundamental part of the individual's world view. When a voodoo curse or spell is cast, the entire community functions in unison and the object of the curse becomes a pariah, separated from his vital emotional lifeline. Often, such an unfortunate person is unable to eat or drink, and despite the fact that no medically identifiable disease state can be found, his bodily systems shut down, causing death. Less dire invocations may produce lesser degrees of illness.

Though Westerners are generally not party to community pressure to the same extent that members of these more traditional societies are, it seems only logical that the mind under severe stress can play an influential role in the production of severe rheumatic disease. It follows that, when the mind is relieved of that distress, the body may heal and return to normal function. You have learned in this book that the mechanism for the production of rheumatic disease is the collection of an excess of immune complexes. In this Filipina there is nothing to suggest that extra antigen was added to start the disease nor any antigen removed to end the disease, so it becomes evident that the cause lies in diminished function of her inflammation defensive systems which in turn are controlled by her brain. Her inadequate inflammation defense may have been due to either inadequate immune phagocytic function or inadequate hypothalamic-cortisol function, or even a combination of each.

The example cited above is an extreme demonstration of how emotional states can influence rheumatic disease, but it is not uncommon to see rheumatic pains accentuated by the different stresses of daily life. One of my patients with mild arthritis became almost immobile with pain whenever her wayward daughter encountered more trouble. Remember that arthritis pain is produced by the summation of several factors.

Currently there is a growing army of non-physicians who are extremely interested in using the power of the mind to control the functions of the body and some of its disease manifestations. At first they were low in profile, but now some university medical researchers as well as researchers at the National Institutes of Health are starting to explore the complexities of the mind and the immune system.

PSYCHONEUROIMMUNOLOGY

Psychoneuroimmunology is the study of the interrelationship of the mind and the immune system and their influences upon the body's health and disease. There is incontrovertible evidence that the mind has the power to create some diseases, including immune diseases like arthritis. Likewise, the mind also has the power to intervene favorably in the progress of some diseases like arthritis.

A principal group of natural chemical agents in this mind-body interaction are called neurotransmitters. Neurotransmitters carry messages not only from one stimulated nerve cell to another, but also from nerves to other kinds of cells, including those that activate glands and muscles. Norepinephrine and serotonin are two well-known chemical transmitters. Decreased supplies of either one can lead to emotional depression. A sense of well-being requires that nerves "talk" to each other regularly. Antidepressant medications are used to overcome severe depression by increasing available supplies of neurotransmitters. In the other direction, excessive amounts of serotonin can trigger hyperexcitive or manic behavior. The brain is the major producer of serotonin. Serotonin is stored in blood platelets and in the lining of the digestive tract. When serotonin is released from platelets at the site of inflammation, it is carried by the blood to the hypothalamus to enable and/or to signal the need for a surge of cortisol, the corticosteroid inhibitor of inflammation.

When a group of Fischer rats, which are bred to be resistant to the development of arthritis for the purpose of being used in scientific research, were given a chemical that blocks the action of cortisol, they all developed arthritis. A similar group of Fischer rats was given a chemical that blocks serotonin, and they too developed arthritis. This information indicates that a neurotransmitter is involved either directly or indirectly in the cortisol control of inflammation. It also suggests that even under normal conditions a subliminal amount of immune complex inflammation is constantly being controlled, even in the complete absence of clinical symptoms of arthritis. Impaired production of some hypothalamic hormones results not only in decreased inflammation control, but it may also produce the tiredness and emotional depression characteristic of arthritis.

The inferences made about the nature of the mind-body relationship are based on clinical observations, but much in the way of hard scientific data is still missing. We are lacking data, for example, on the exact mode of influence of stress upon the activity of the white blood cells, though receptor sites for neurotransmitters have been found on lymphocytes and macrophages, strongly suggesting an interaction between the mind and the immune system. It is clear that immune response is depressed as the result of stress and that the body becomes more susceptible to disease as a result, but it is not at all clear exactly what nerve and chemical pathways are involved in the brain-immune process.

BIOCHEMICALS AND THE BRAIN

It is no coincidence, I believe, that a biochemical factor that makes an excess of immune complexes for producing arthritis can simultaneously produce adverse alterations of the mind for the same reason. One patient of mine—we will call her Diane B #43—serves as an excellent demonstration of this connection.

Twenty-eight when I first saw her, Diane had had pains from rheumatoid arthritis for many years. She also had great difficulty verbally expressing herself, being unable to finish sentences, so much so that she could make but limited sense. Over the years, psychiatrists and psychologists had declared her to be mentally impaired and permanently unemployable.

Then I put Diane through the usual drill with nutrition. The Food Elimination Diet not only removed most of her arthritis pain, but she also gained normal, intelligent speech. We found the offending agent to be caffeine. Harder to accomplish was the task of undoing the low self-esteem which she had developed as the result of so many years of self-helplessness, which was reinforced by her psychologists. She had to be convinced that she was now capable of enjoying a normal life. Happily, she was able to make that adjustment and today she remains healthy and productive.

Your Conscious Brain and Your Subconscious Hypothalamus

The subconscious hypothalamus with its surrounding limbic area is a primitive part of the brain; it controls basic functions such as temperature and blood pressure, and basic emotions such as sexuality, fear and rage. The hypothalamus is also part of your memory data bank in which your experiential attitudes lie hidden in "tape recordings" which are played regularly to your conscious brain. Your hypothalamic functions are automatic in nature.

The larger, conscious part of your brain, the part that is believed to separate humans from lower animals, is where you do most of your thinking. This too can be influenced at times by both good and bad emotional "tapes." Countless nerves maintain a constant intercommunication between the conscious and the subconscious brain.

Many women with premenstrual tension say angry or cruel words to family and friends while menstruating and then apologize later. They would truly like to immediately curtail such improper actions, but their subconscious hypothalamus is so severely irritated by menstrually-associated immune complexes that the basic hypothalamic emotions override any conscious control. This exemplifies the subconscious actually taking control over the conscious.

With biofeedback we can learn to increase skin temperature in the hands and fingers by concentratedly thinking about warming them, literally diverting blood flow to the hands through an act of will. This finger warming represents the conscious mind taking over a failed function of the subconscious, a skill worth mastering for persons whose cold fingers resulting from Raynaud's disease can be especially uncomfortable. Biofeedback is also designed to give patients audible evidence of the degree of electrical activity they can still generate in a paralyzed limb, an important step in helping them to retrain their muscles to act again.

There are times when it is important to reprogram a troublemaking subconscious hypothalamus, but how do we get to the center of our brain to do that? We fill the conscious brain, over which we have direct control through eyes and ears, with reconstructive data that will be shared at least partly with the hypothalamus. If one repeatedly, with relaxation and audiotapes, accesses the subconscious hypothalamus with messages for healing and suggestions for new behaviors, a subconscious drive for the solution of a particular problem may possibly be established. This can be reinforced by programs of daily positive thinking. Hypnosis and self-hypnosis are also used to break through the screen of conscious interference so that a more reliable hypothalamic imprint may be affected.

As an example of an imprint, cancer patients are frequently taught to create a picture in their minds of an army of voracious macrophages eating up their cancer cells. The conscious development of subconscious visualizations has often been effective in controlling rheumatic disease.

In some ways, this is similar to the placebo effect—a significant symptomatic improvement gained from faith, trust and mental manipulation. Once pooh-poohed, we now know it to be a genuine player in some recoveries. But we should learn to harness the power of the spirit, which will at times yield amazing visible and symptomatic improvements. Such powers have repeatedly superseded many modern measures of medicine and surgery.

Influences of Stress Upon Immune Function

Research has shown that stressed monkeys have a reduced number of immune T-lymphocytes with which to fight disease. Stressed human beings also present lowered immune response under similar conditions. Emotional stress is commonly known to increase the symptoms of arthritis. When we combine the meanings of these three sentences, we would say that arthritis can be made *worse* by depressing immune function. It is important to remember that one of the objectives of modern rheumatic therapy is to *decrease* the potency of the immune system with agents such as methotrexate. Their approach is, of course, directly contrary to my own view.

The rheumatic therapy that I recommend, and the only one that seems logical when one considers the role of stress in arthritis, is to *increase* the power of the immune system. Stress-linked immune depression certainly is not limited to just what has been observed in the lymphocytes. Theory says that the lymphatic depression alone would result in reduced antibody production, which in turn makes a reduced number of immune complexes, and which ultimately should reduce inflammation; *but* the combined three sentences tell us that is exactly opposite to what happens clinically with stress. Immune depression of the lymphocytes in all likelihood is accompanied by immune depression of the phagocytes. Though I know of no medical attempt to prove this key phagocytic factor, the surrounding circumstances mandate its reality. You already well know that decreased phagocytosis results in increased immune complexes and in increased pain and inflammation.

Stress also reduces the output of neurotransmitters, which in turn could limit the action of the cells of the defensive immune system and also diminish the cortisol inflammation protection by the hypothalamus. Logical arthritis therapy would avoid stress and try to promote the subconscious hypothalamus so that natural defenses could function maximally.

The immune system was devised to help us live long and well. The most logical approach to the control of rheumatic disease is to enhance that protective system, not destroy it. My natural approach in therapy is to strengthen and assist the immune system so that it can function optimally, and also to relieve that system as much as reasonable of its antigenic burden. The therapeutic destruction of the immune system should be reserved for last-ditch heroics in trading life for a limited period of reduced pain from a devastating disease, but only when nothing else of a safer nature has helped.

Stress is Your Interpretation of Events

Psychological stress is not limited to the details of what a person actually experiences, but also includes that person's perception or interpretation of that experience—what does it mean to him. Perceptions may be influenced by the correctness of related information and also by attitudes of bias, faith, paranoia, etc, that become part of the mind's internal dialogue. Every ball game has happy winners and sad losers, though they all saw the same event.

Psychological stress management deals with conducting your life in a manner which avoids some stresses, and learning how to cope more effectively with stress factors that are unavoidable.

Courses in stress management as well as in assertiveness training all have the potential to give you new and better tools for living more comfortably within your skin. Support groups formed by people with similar difficulties and experiences can assist in helping the individual deal with adverse realities that are essentially unchangeable. They attempt to substitute a sense of empowerment and control for the sense of helplessness that existed before. Such groups often work wonders, helping fibromyalgia patients cope with their pain, helping alcoholics adopt new lifestyles, extending life expectancy for breast cancer survivors, and assisting children with chronic diseases to rise above their handicaps. All of these processes of therapy require your very active participation and commitment. You must convince yourself that you can do it, and then harness that *mind power* to achieve specific goals. The power is there, if you are willing to uncover it and to readjust your mind-talk toward positive rather than negative expectations.

One positive expectation you want to work on if you are hampered by sickness is that you can be healthy again. When you relinquish your mind power to a state of weak helplessness, your chances for recovery are diminished. Feelings of helplessness and loss of control are well established to be the most damaging of attitudes for performance of the body as a whole, and for the performance of the immune system in particular. Olympic sportsmen, who have abilities that far exceed the ordinary person, must get psyched up in order to give their ultimate, supreme performance. In the daily sport of life and death, you must get psyched up in order to outdo the enemy of disease.

Your conscious mind supplies the doorway for introducing new and healthier ideas into your subconscious hypothalamus, where they can be stored in your natural computer. Sometimes, when the conscious brain is resistant to new ideas, that barrier may be overcome by the use of hypnosis. Hypnosis can't make you do what you do not want to do, but it might implant suggestions which, after some conscious-subconscious mind-talk, might be at least partly accepted. Therapy sessions with a psychological counselor, or repeated playing of therapeutic tapes may etch new and more positive attitudes into your hypothalamus; and once there, you can subconsciously play them back for constructive solutions when your body is under siege.

The subconscious hypothalamus maintains the ideal functions in a happy brain-body, while it adversely alters function in the depressed brain-body, such as stimulating the stomach to acid ulceration and depressing the immune system. Your autonomic (automatic) nervous system and neurotransmitters make up the communication system between the brain and the physical body for many of these reactions.

The brain that has been subjected to a constant influx of emotional insults and stress produces fewer neurotransmitters. Reduced neurotransmitters produce feelings of depression, loss of appetite, difficulty sleeping and reduced sexual drive. Most modern medicines for depression function by increasing the effective amount of your neurotransmitters. People with rheumatic disease commonly experience poor sleeping and depression, and it is no surprise that the neurotransmitter medicines also help solve those two problems plus reducing a little of your pain.

I believe that at least a small portion of my success in the treatment of rheumatic disease arises from my putting patients in control of the management of their own disease. I tell each patient that I will teach them and train them, with the assistance of written information and guide sheets, to be their own day-to-day arthritis doctor; and, at the end of the instruction period, when they are performing well, I verbally confer upon them the degree of "Doctor of your own arthritis." They assume the responsibility of looking after their own problem, particularly with prednisone—the what, when and how much to use. This management is designed to change their role of helpless victims of a terrible disease to that of being captain of their ship. My advice is always available when requested by telephone (from physicians only) or by visit.

HEALING ENERGIES FROM TOUCH

The chiropractor is not held in high esteem by most members of the medical profession. This is largely because the chiropractor's working hypothesis is that disease arises from interference with normal nerve function traceable to spinal misalignment. Following this line of thinking, treatment relies upon manipulation and adjustment of the spinal column to restore normal nerve function. Even though I am not in agreement with some of their hypotheses, I have no doubt that the chiropractor has the ability to make many patients more comfortable when physicians have failed.

One therapeutic modality that the chiropractor uses that the physician routinely omits is the laying on of hands, the establishing of physical contact with the skin of each and every patient. That this is effective in creating a healing environment has been shown over and over again: babies are soothed by gentle handling, and they have thrived better in foundling homes where volunteers come in and just hold them in their arms. A Chinese therapist has very significantly relieved fibrocystic disease by hand massage. There are several groups of alternative healing therapists who obtain favorable results by touching troubled areas or by touching skin reference points for disease in remote organs or tissues.

I believe, as do holistic doctors, that patients at appropriate times should be touched and hugged, and I have held the hands of thousands of women at the time of their physical and emotional stresses. There are positive healing energies that are transferred or released by touch, or perhaps by merely entering the aura that closely surrounds us all, without actually touching. Those spiritual energies seem to be transmitted to, and at least temporarily stored in, the subconscious hypothalamus for a favorable influence upon how the body feels and functions. Unfortunately, Western mores and Western medicine look askance upon a doctor who holds the hands of his women patients, and he is all but pilloried if he holds the hands of his male patients. MDs who present themselves as holistic physicians are sometimes treated as non-members of The Club! Just a few days ago I was stopped on the street by a woman who wanted to tell me how pleased she was when I held her hand forty years ago as she labored with her baby.

HYPOTHALAMIC FUNCTION IN IMMUNE DISEASE

The hypothalamus is not part of the immune system, though there are many close interactions. The subconscious hypothalamus functions not only as part of the mind, but it also controls the function of many tissues and glands, as well as having its own hormone production. The hypothalamus is discussed in some detail in this chapter not only because it is inseparably interwoven with immune function and inflammation, but also because its functions can be intentionally modified to your benefit by several modes of psychological intervention. Perhaps the production of cortisol sounds unrelated to your mind-talk, but actually by favorably altering adverse mind-talk to peaceful mind-talk, you can improve its cortisol responses. If you understand about hypothalamic function, you will have a firmer grasp on the realities of what you can accomplish by improving your conscious-subconscious dialogue.

Science moderately understands hypothalamic management of cortisol production for arthritis control. The biochemical messengers Interleukin-1 and neurotransmitters are released from the site of inflammation to go tell the hypothalamus to get busy. But we do not yet understand very well how stress and depression actually diminish immune function. Reducing neurotransmitters could reduce activation of immune white cells that have neurotransmitter receptor sites.

People with arthritis have an inadequate hypothalamic response to stress. I believe this occurs as the result of the hypothalamus being rapidly fatigued by a constant bombardment of messages to make more cortisol in response to inflammation. The occurrence of fatigue is good, because it prevents the hypothalamus from producing an excess of cortisol; but it is also bad, because it allows inflammation and resulting pain to continue unabated. If the hypothalamus did not switch off, then a large portion of the arthritic population would be moon-faced and manifest those even more serious problems of excess cortisol.

When prednisone is used according to the Microdose System described in Chapter Seven, important things occur: total inflammation is artificially reduced while the hypothalamus is rested periodically for recuperation. When recovered, the hypothalamus is returned to normal function until it is again depressed by excessive messages for action. The intermittent hypothalamic function in place of constant depression by either constant messengers or constant prednisone is why the Microdose prednisone obtains markedly improved results over the much larger, continuous doses of standard therapy.

How hypothalamic recuperation works on the patient's behalf is demonstrated by the case of Marcia S #25, whom I introduced in Chapter 7. You will remember that Marcia came to me after suffering with osteoarthritis for nine years. With prednisone induction she brought her pain score of 36 down to zero. Since her pain score rarely rose from this position, she repeated Microdose prednisone only once every two or three months.

During the continuous display of arthritis symptoms Marcia had known earlier, we can reasonably assume that her hypothalamus suffered from constant depression. Under Microdose therapy she went for many weeks without medication and without pain. We can reasonably assume that during those many painless weeks that the hypothalamus was working perfectly. When some additional complexes increased the immune complex load above the ability of the anti-inflammatory defense to hold it in check, she would need a few days of prednisone to regain the upper hand. The sooner she responded with prednisone, the easier it was to keep her problem in check. Her average daily intake of prednisone averaged only 0.4 mg! I would like to introduce the possibility that if Marcia were to approach her problem with techniques of relaxation, self-hypnosis and meditation to enhance her hypothalamic function, that she might no longer need the tiny amounts of prednisone.

HYPOTHALAMIC ENHANCEMENT BY B12

We have previously pictured the way in which phagocytes are made more active with large vitamin supplements. Vital amines, or vitamins, are chemicals required by all cells of the body for proper metabolic function, and it is reasonable to assume that the nerves of the depressed hypothalamus could also obtain enhanced function from vitamin supplementation.

The case of Monica T #44 shows how helpful vitamins can be in this regard. Monica was 74 years old when she first consulted me, having suffered from osteoarthritis and fibromyalgia for the previous ten years. For several years she also had almost complete urinary incontinence which required her to wear absorbent padding. No previous measures of therapy had been effective for either problem.

Monica's baseline total pain score was 110. Prednisone and the FED had no beneficial effects. But, when I began vitamin B12 shots, she not only had the pain score drop to 70, but she also regained control of her bladder. Thereafter, spironolactone saw Monica's pain score rapidly sliding down past 53. Not surprisingly, her mood also improved greatly.

The possible connection between the B12 shots and regained bladder control may lie in the control center for regulating the urinary bladder, which is located in the hypothalamus; but I cannot determine that for sure, because it is also possible that the benefit came from local nerve improvement, or even both. Gary C #14 also had his intestinal function returned to normal by B12, and this I cautiously attribute to another control center in the hypothalamus specific to intestinal motility. I have found that vitamin B12 has repeatedly demonstrated an ability to improve bladder function, intestinal function, arthritis pain and mood through its possible influence upon the hypothalamus. I believe it is reasonable to consider that this same array of symptoms could be at least partly ameliorated through psychological adjustments that could improve mind-talk and happiness of the subconscious mind-body. When we go to war on disease, it is best to have all reasonably positive factors working for us—do not rely upon one weapon alone.

YOUR STATE OF MIND/YOUR DISEASE

Patients with Multiple Personality Disorders (MPD) have been known to exhibit different health and illness patterns depending upon the specific personality they were "inhabiting." As one personality changes into another, as with flipping an electrical switch, so may the disease states with which they are linked. We have seen this in manifestations of hypertension, epilepsy, warts, rashes, allergies, night blindness and diabetes. The changing of personality concerns nothing more than a shift of gears in the same biochemical apparatus—nothing added, nothing subtracted—but the function of the mind switches.

Take as an example, a young boy with MPD who would manifest an allergy to orange juice by breaking out in hives with one persona, but would show no such symptoms with orange juice in another persona. The only apparent change that was made was the brain attitude. One possible way to explain this would be that the hypothalamus was blocked from functioning and unable to control the inflammatory response in one persona, and then became unblocked in the next persona and able to perform its normal anti-inflammatory CRF functions.

A similar brain inhibition was demonstrated in the case of a sensitized patient who, under hypnosis and with suggestion, received a tuberculin injection, to which she was normally reactive, and manifested no immune response. These radical metabolic and immune switches of MPD and hypnosis confound the minds of conventionally-trained physicians, but evidence is there to prove it can happen. It shows once again that if you are strong enough to control your brain, you can take control of your health, arthritis included!

Try this curious example of Pavlovian training for another piece of evidence regarding the interplay of sensory experience and health: A group of laboratory animals was repeatedly treated with a medicine that suppressed the immune system response, and with each treatment they were simultaneously exposed to the taste of saccharine-sweetened water. Another group of laboratory animals was repeatedly treated with a medicine that enhanced the immune system response, and, each time they were treated, they were simultaneously exposed to the smell of camphor. Neither saccharine nor camphor ordinarily affects the immune reaction; but, when the immune-altering medicines were withdrawn, the saccharine group still experienced immune depression with the taste of saccharine and the camphor group still experienced immune enhancement with the smell of camphor.

The immune systems of each group had learned to alter their function in response to the associated brain stimulations of taste and smell.

The principles of the above animal experimentation have had a direct, practical, human application. A child in a Cleveland children's hospital, who was suffering from lupus, required a very toxic drug which had the characteristic of producing severe side effects. Each time the toxic drug was administered to the child, it was mixed with cod liver oil for a strong taste and was accompanied by a strong smell of rose perfume. Over the course of time, as the dose of the drug was gradually diminished, the child's body continued to respond just as well to the reduced drug dosage, which was still accompanied by the taste and the scent, as though it were getting the full dosage. This allowed good, effective therapy with a reduced dosage and fewer side effects. I suspect that if adult patients were to be told of such a scheme (informed consent) for themselves, the power of the beneficial delusion would be lost.

The main principle for you to learn from the related anecdotes is that actual functions of the body can be controlled or altered by simply changing the attitudes of your mind or by the introduction of meaningful data into the mind. Usually you must play an active part in slowly reconstructing the functioning patterns of your mind.

EDGAR CAYCE, A MESSENGER FOR THE COSMIC SPIRIT

Edgar Cayce, an American who lived from 1877 to 1945, was a charismatic healer strongly oriented to the Bible and Christianity. He had limited public schooling and no medical training whatsoever. However, in 30,000 psychic trances he supplied information that made possible the diagnosis and treatment of countless seriously ill patients, many of whom had been unresponsive to standard medical care. While in a trance, he would use medical terms and give advice that he himself could not comprehend when he was fully awake. Many people believe that Cayce performed this "impossible feat" as a speaker for the benevolent Cosmic Spirit of God. In spite of reportedly excellent medical therapeutic results obtained by hundreds of patients who followed the advice of his psychic readings, Cayce was abused, shunned and discredited by the medical community.

Many of his patients suffered from arthritis. A representative example of his extraordinary insight is contained in the report of a 1932 reading in which Cayce undertook the care of an 18-year-old woman with severely stiff, swollen and disabling arthritis over much of her body. Though she was unresponsive to standard medical care, Cayce's recommendations were successful. Among the recommendations Cayce cited for her: selective diet (exogenous allergens), points of infection (bacterial allergens), and adrenal and other glandular function (endogenous, autoimmune hormone allergens). He also recommended therapy to the lacteal duct area (enhancing the immune system).

I am personally awed that more than fifty years ago Cayce, in his role as a non-physician speaker for the Cosmic Spirit, was able to outline most of the essential and new principles which I am teaching you today for the management of your arthritis. None of Cayce's effective therapies were accepted by organized medicine, so in the intervening years more than one hundred million Americans have suffered unnecessarily from the ravages of arthritis. I believe Cayce was empowered by the Benevolent Spirit to help mankind, but mankind did not have ears to hear fifty years ago. I pray, but am still not certain, that mankind will have ears to hear my message today— and gain the powers of that Healing Spirit.

I at least want to suggest that you consider adopting the concept of the spirit of the God of your understanding with a devoted and meditating mind so that your mind-talk can be most rewarding.

MEDITATION AND THE MIND

Many thousands of year ago, shamans and other wise men worked on the concept of a close relationship between body and mind. This belief was more prominent in Eastern than in Western cultures and that separation is still manifested in both religious and medical viewpoints today. Easterners in particular regard meditation as a doorway to enlightenment, and systems such as yoga began in India long before the Christian era.

Deepak Chopra, M.D., an Indian himself, swings toward the Eastern concept in his program of Quantum Healing, which he defines as the ability of one mode of consciousness, the mind, to correct the mistakes in another mode of consciousness, the body. This ability, he says, works through an ''intelligence'' in every single cell of the body, the intelligence being carried by its DNA; he also believes that our billions of cells with their DNA intelligence act as one unit.

Eastern philosophers and healers believe that spirituality extends beyond our ordinary three states of awake-asleep-dreaming into a fourth stage, which can be reached through proper meditation. The spirituality could be assigned to either a Supreme Being or to an extension of the Spirit of the Self. Meditation brings the mind out of its ordinary boundaries of consciousness, and in the process alters many aspects of physiological function. The rate of oxygen consumption by the body is a measure of the intensity of body function. In the state of sleep the body uses 10 percent less oxygen than in the state of being awake. The oxygen consumption in hypnosis is about the same as being awake. Meditation can bring the rate down as much as 18 percent. These findings of a depressed body functional state in meditation are supported by the skin electric reaction and the blood lactate levels. These physiological changes brought about by meditation are not the benefits, but the evidence of its having occurred, evidence that goes beyond or transcends the conscious disconnection of sleep.

Meditation is best practiced in a place where there are no distractions, where you can comfortably assume a meditative posture, where you can focus your attention on a meaningless thing like your breathing or by making some repetitive sound like *Om*, and when you can assume a passive, receptive attitude with a mind that has been essentially emptied of active or controversial thoughts. You may receive imperceptible information or guidance from the spirit world or Cosmic Spirit while you are in that state of openmindedness. Meditation should be practiced once or twice a day for 20 minutes or so.

This meditation practice is sometimes called Transcendental Meditation, or TM. Through the use of meditation one can reach a state of greater relaxation, decreased anxiety and a greater sense of well-being. There may be an associated reduction of headaches, chronic immune ailments, colds and allergies, and improved sleep. Meditation creates an increased awareness of your surroundings, yet reduces the potential for inappropriate anxiety about them. It may bring control over a wandering and distracted mind.

Robert Wallace, Ph.D. demonstrated by observations of human blood pressure, hearing and vision that those who regularly practiced meditation were functionally five to ten years younger than those who did not meditate.

Dr. Chopra tells about a patient who was diagnosed with a large brain cancer on the basis not only of symptoms, but by X-ray and by biopsy as well. The patient elected meditation as his therapy rather than the apparently hopeless surgery, radiation or chemotherapy. Six months later a medical checkup detected no signs whatsoever of the tumor!

Doctor Chopra also writes about a 35-year-old woman who had breast cancer. Surgery removed her breast and also found spread of the cancer to her armpit. Then another cancer in the other breast required removal of that second breast. She experienced a poor response to chemotherapy. At age 38 she delivered a baby successfully, but she was sick from active cancer and from bone pain caused by the cancer which had spread there. With her life expectancy poor at best, she began transcendental meditation followed by Ayurvedic treatment using the primordial sound technique. As her bone pain rapidly declined, X-rays indicated the cancer had gone into total remission. Her abnormal blood chemistries also returned to a normal range. She is still pain-free and emotionally at peace.

The purpose of citing these clinical examples is to demonstrate to you the factual possibility of controlling your bodily functions, such as the immune reactivity involved in your arthritis, by enlisting the power and the full cooperative support of your mind and of your God. This would not necessarily be a primary therapy of choice for rheumatic disease, but it might make your future brighter by making it a member of your full therapeutic team for arthritis. At least catalog it in your memory, because some day you may want to draw upon it.

Regardless of how you apply mind therapy—through positive thinking, the laying-on of hands, hypnosis or meditation—it is usually a slow process, requiring many repetitions for etching new pathways of performance into the brain. At least once a day give yourself a reminder session to facilitate internalization of the therapeutic thoughts and messages. Don't be dismayed if you have to wait weeks or sometimes months before you detect the first tangible, physical benefits, and even those positive signs will represent only the beginning of your efforts. The new highways of thought, behavior and bodily response will continue to need maintenance, just as serious athletes must persist in physical conditioning throughout their careers. There are no guarantees of success, of course, but you have a good chance of having the symptoms of your rheumatic disease subdued, and you will almost certainly develop a more tranquil, healthy attitude about the multiple stresses of your life, which in turn may lead to a more pleasant life with fewer illnesses and a greater duration. Remember that meditation is designed not only to cure your problem diseases both large and small, but also to maintain a healthy and longer life. You cannot lose by trying!

REMEMBER

1. Psychoneuroimmunology is the study of the interrelationship of the mind and the immune system and their influence upon the body's health and disease.
2. There is incontrovertible evidence that the mind has the power to create some diseases, including immune diseases like arthritis. Likewise, the mind has the power to intervene favorably in the progress of some diseases, including arthritis.
3. Your hypothalamus is the basic manager of bodily function. When stressed or irritated, it can lead to malfunction and disease.
4. Stress *increases* arthritis pain by *depressing* the immune system. Modern arthritis medical theory and therapy also depress immunity.
5. Stress can be modified by various forms of stress management

including a counselor, support groups, hypnotherapy and by oneself.

6. Positive, disease-fighting imagery may help your immune system fight disease.
7. Touching one another is a modality for transmitting positive energies for physical and emotional comfort and healing.
8. Meditation may transcend your ordinary states of consciousness and may enhance brain and immune function.
9. Contacting the Cosmic Spirit may enhance brain-controlled health and tranquility.
10. Complete arthritis therapy requires removal of antigens and supports for the defensive systems as well as spiritual mind control.

13
Physical Therapy and Exercise

YOU CANNOT RUN ARTHRITIS OUT OF TOWN!

It HAS been established beyond a shadow of doubt that regular physical exercise is good for your general health. Covert Bailey has stated, "If exercise could be packaged in a pill it would be the most heavily prescribed medicine in history."

Exercise is very important for people with rheumatic disease in order to maintain their general state of good health. However, I believe that ordinary exercise is not significantly effective in the treatment of the inflammation and pains of the basic, specific immune disease itself. Ordinary exercise does not alter the supply of antigens for immune complexes, nor does it significantly alter the defensive power of the anti-inflammatory systems. In fact, excessive exercise or physical work seems to rather reliably increase the total daily pain score for the majority of patients, and that increase may include joints that had zero pain at the beginning of the exercise. It would seem that there is a happy medium between inactivity and too much exercise, and I would judge that to be about ten or twenty minutes daily for gently exercising your comfortable or just mildly uncomfortable joints.

A study of 5,000 college women by Harvard University has revealed that those sportswomen who participated with teams for two or more years experienced only one-third the incidence of reproductive tract cancers as did the other college women and only half the number of breast cancers. There was also a similar reduction of benign tumors of the genital tract and breasts of these sportswomen. It is open to conjecture as to whether the benefit of reduced tumor formation is representative of an enhanced immune system which was enabled to destroy tumors upon their inception or whether this represents a reduced ovarian production of antigenic native progesterone which would no longer be able to stimulate normal reproductive tract tissues into a neoplastic or cancerous transformation. To my knowledge, there was not a simultaneous determination of the relative incidence of rheumatic disease, but I suspect that a parallel relationship would be found.

It has been determined that women who have used oral contraceptives (inhibition of native progesterone) experience a 50 percent reduction in the incidence of rheumatoid arthritis. My answer for this improved rheumatic status, which otherwise has had no good scientific explanation, is that the hormonal medication either inhibits the production of native progesterone or successfully competes with it at the progesterone receptor sites of the potential antigenic protein so that the native progesterone is removed from the arena of the potential immune reactivity. By thus removing native progesterone from having contact with the immune system, there is a reduction of the time exposure which is usually necessary for the immune system to first learn to be reactive to the native progesterone and then to increase its reactivity step by step through repeated monthly exposures. This will result in decreasing the total of tissue irritation and inflammation which has the potential of transforming normal gynecic tissue into abnormal fibroids or cancer. It is usually difficult to find a woman with fibroids who does not also have some added feature of menstrually-associated pain, bleeding, edema or premenstrual tension (autoimmune irritation). The influence of the excessive conditioning required to be successful at team sports for women is that it tends to inhibit ovulation and its associated production of native progesterone. Such women often fail to menstruate during the time of their intense training.

By the time that you have developed rheumatic disease, it is possibly too late on your biological clock to create a significant difference in deep-rooted disease, particularly when your attempt to become athletic can be strongly hindered by uncomfortable joint disease. My own personal severe increase of rheumatic disease occurred in spite of the fact that I had been jogging several miles almost daily for several years, was playing tennis one evening a week, and doing 25 to 50 push-ups daily. I still exercise at home mildly every day, but no longer as the athlete I cannot be.

In specific and beneficial relationship to the arthritis patient, exercise maintains better bone strength, inhibits the adhesion of inflamed joint surfaces, and can stretch out and normalize the range of motion for joints and tendons that have been previously scarred by old rheumatic inflammation. Examples of this rehabilitation can be seen in cases #29 LV and #30 MK, in which the complete therapeutic turn-off of inflammation allowed healing and then rehabilitation by exercise of the feet. Repetitive exercise does not relieve the inflammatory pains and swelling, but tends to aggravate and accentuate them. I believe that pain is built into our bodies as a warning signal: Retreat, stay away! Accordingly, my recommendation is that exercising be done within the limits of reasonable comfort. Move your joints to the fringes of discomfort, but do not keep pushing the joint through your zone of discomfort. I do suggest that at least once a day and possibly twice each day you try, within your reasonable tolerance of pain, to put your painful joint through its full range of motion. There is to be just one such excursion of the painful joint, and this is intended to prevent the possible adhesion of the inflamed joint surfaces. More activity than that might be damaging to the joint. Repetitive motions and true exercise for that ailing joint must be reserved until that inflammatory process has been overcome by an effective means of immune complex reduction. When it comes time to stretch out a joint previously limited in range of motion by inflammation which has now been eliminated, stretch it gently two or three times daily. Local heat, such as with a heating pad or a hot water soak, seems to assist in the stretching. Gentle day-after-day persistence will gain you much more than one episode of violent insistence.

When you start your gentle exercising, go at it slowly for just a few minutes at first. Make it a routine part of the beginning of each day. Devise your own system of exercises that will move every joint from head to toe, and add them one by one. Rather than doing your exercising at a club or spa, do it at home, where it will cost you nothing, where inclement weather cannot stop you on any day, and where you will not feel obliged to do more than your body wants to do because other people are watching you. The aim of exercise is to make you a healthy and mobile person, not a super-athletic person.

Walking a mile each day is a universally accepted health measure, as long as your walking joints do not hurt. If your home has a flight of stairs, it will supply controlled cardiac stress without the need to run.

A 30-year-old laborer, patient Randy N #45, sustained fractures and third degree burns in an auto accident in 1980. The right shoulder was stapled and the left shoulder was broken also. Skin grafting was necessary for the burns. In 1983 he developed a pain in his right shoulder which was investigated by arthroscopy and then the rotator cuff was repaired again. He fell at work again in 1984, making it necessary to repair the right rotator cuff still once more. Since that last repair he has had a painful and weak right shoulder and arm in spite of persistent physical therapy with heat and massage, and with weight-lifting exercises through the full but painful range of motion. A cortisone shot in the shoulder had been of minimal help. He experienced flares of pain from once a week to once a month. There was an associated difficulty in sleeping.

Randy's total pain score was 5 to 6 in the right shoulder only. I reduced the physical therapy to heat and massage without any motion. A prednisone induction brought the pain score down to 1, and the score was maintained at zero to 1 with Microdose prednisone. After the pain score was zero for about ten days, we started passive (assisted) full range of motion, then active full range of motion, and then, finally, to gradual and gentle lightly weighted motion. Full comfort was the mandatory guideline for each step of the way. The average use of maintenance prednisone was 2 mg per day. At the end of eight weeks the surprised physical therapist found Randy's arm to be three times stronger than at the beginning, and he was ready to return to work. The suspicions of his being a Workmen's Compensation malingerer disappeared. Ten months later the comfort and strength were being maintained with occasional use of Microdose prednisone therapy.

There are two separate aspects of this success story. First is the proper cyclic use of prednisone to bring the basic inflammation under control. Second is the limitation of joint motion to what is comfortable. Under the auspices of comfort, the progress was very rapid. If you were to sprain your ankle, the ordinary medical advice for the best results would be to rest your ankle until comfortable and healed. It does not make good sense to give the opposite recommendations for arthritic joints.

Heat, massage, diathermy, galvanic therapy, magnetic field therapy and other such modalities of local therapy all seem to have a common ability to relax and reduce the pain of the affected area of inflammation. Improved circulation and improved cellular function are the rational explanation for the improvements attained. Unfortunately, if there is a continuing immune irritation, the improvements tend to be only of a temporary nature that may last hours, days or weeks until repeat physical therapy is required. Such relief, though temporary, is warmly welcomed by those in severe pain. Lasting results are to be obtained only by reducing or eliminating the source and the activity of immune complexes. I believe, because many of my patients found through experience, that the chiropractic doctor who manipulates gently is often of great help in making rheumatic joints feel better. This again is a welcomed, temporary relief, but it holds no element of cure for rheumatic disease.

Chinese acupuncture has been applied to all sorts of bodily and mental conditions, including arthritis, for thousands of years. Acupuncture concerns a system of many hundreds of points on the skin which have been very carefully mapped out anatomically and which theoretically have a nerve connection with the function and sensation of some remote organ or tissue. A combination of needles is then inserted at those skin points that control the area or organ which is in trouble. Additional stimulation for increased effect may be accomplished by twirling the needle in place or by adding an electrical stimulus. The experienced Chinese have claimed, and also have demonstrated, some absolutely astounding acupuncture results, such as doing a gastrectomy under acupuncture anesthesia with the patient wide awake and talking during the operation. However, the Western medical community has been very slow to be convinced. My patients who have been treated by acupuncture report that there has been little or no benefit obtained from such treatments. It is likely that those who responded very well to acupuncture would have no need to seek my services as well. I cannot believe that acupuncture can stop the production of immune complexes, though I can understand that great faith on the part of the patient can have very significant influences through the function of the hypothalamic region of the brain. This aspect is considered in more detail in Chapter 12.

There is a Western offshoot of acupuncture called reflexology. This system follows the same zonal mapping of the body as does acupuncture, but the skin points of concern are treated by finger pressure and deep rubbing for several minutes. Other objects may be used for point or regional pressure, such as combs, rubber bands, clamps, clothespins, clenching teeth, yawning and even a "magic massager." My book learning and brief clinical exposure to reflexology leave me in great doubt about its validity.

There is an ancient Chinese system for establishing and maintaining mental and physical health called Tai Chi, which I believe is an attractive proposition for rheumatic people. This health system incorporates the combination of meditation and gentle physical exercise. A brief period of meditation is recommended for each day. The daily physical exercise is designed to activate the flow of impeded healing energies throughout the body. The concept is that natural body energies are supplemented with extra energy withdrawn from the earth below and from a string or cone of energy which extends through the very top of your head. The exercises are formulated to increase the influx of outside energy and to direct it to troubled tissues. The claimed results are the increase of muscular strength, the directed healing of unwell tissues, and the establishment of mental quietude. The exercises do not entail full extension or flexion of joints, do not use weighted objects, do not require speed, and do not stress the cardiovascular and respiratory systems. It is unlikely that you will sweat or breathe hard. No joint is to be moved if that gentle flow of motion elicits more than minimal pain or discomfort. The concept is that your painful joints will benefit from the improved health of the rest of your body and that they will benefit and heal from the improved flow of energies through your body and through your troubled points. This system is easy to learn, easy to do, and has reputedly helped many people with arthritis. I note with special interest their specific recommendation: *do not hurt* the joints by painful motion.

Relatively unweighted, passive exercise can be obtained by going into a swimming pool where your arms, legs and body weigh almost nothing, because of the buoyancy of the water. There you can more easily work your arms and legs without stress, but always be sure to keep your motions within a comfortable range. The pool is primarily for gentle exercise, not for swimming. A heated pool is distinctly more comfortable and relaxing to your tense muscles. Hot tubs are good as long as you keep your body submerged in the shallow water for its buoyancy as well as the relaxing heat.

Most rheumatic people find that the longer they are inactive, the stiffer and more uncomfortable they become. Even when reading an exciting book, they will periodically get up to stretch their uncomfortable muscles. When these same people go to bed, they vainly hope to have eight hours of sound, undisturbed sleep; but, the longer they are inactively lying in bed, and regardless of the consistency of the bed, the more uncomfortable they become. Most rheumatic people, but not all, find that their total pain score is distinctly worse each morning as they get out of bed. That is why I recommend that you do your scoring about a quarter to a half hour or so later, after you have had a chance to stretch out a little.

There are advertisements by sadistic mattress manufacturers everywhere about getting yourself an orthopedic mattress to improve your back pains. Such mattresses are "scientifically firm and supportive." It is also frequently advised that a wide, flat board be placed under your mattress for "support." When my back was hurting severely, I fell victim to such TV advice by buying the "best" hard bed and discarding my lovely soft one. I felt unhappy and duped with the change; and, when I checked with my patients, the almost unanimous answer was that they too were sorry, because they had forfeited a comfortable, soft old friend for no advantage to their rheumatic backs.

I advise that, if you are awakened at night by back or joint pains, do not stay under the nice warm covers, else you will writhe sleeplessly for the rest of the night. Get out of bed and do your loosening-up exercises. Even though more fully awake, you can then get back to a comfortable sleep more easily. In the morning do not follow the trail to your mattress man, but follow the directions for immune control as outlined in this book. My opinion is that it generally makes no difference whether you buy hard or soft mattresses—just suit your own personal desires for sleeping comfort. You will do better to spend your mattress money on controlling your immune complexes.

REMEMBER

1. Exercise is good for your general health.
2. Exercise should not involve joints that are painful.
3. There is little to suggest that exercise will control immune complex irritation, while there is much to suggest that it increases pain scores.
4. The objective of exercise for rheumatic people is to maintain a reasonable range of comfortable joint motion and a mild to moderate muscular strength.
5. Stressful cardiorespiratory aerobic exercises, although good for your body, can sometimes be counterproductive for arthritic joints.
6. After immune inflammation has been conquered by other immune complex-controlling measures, more stressful joint exercising may be in order.
7. I believe the consistency of your mattress has little to do with your rheumatic back pains.

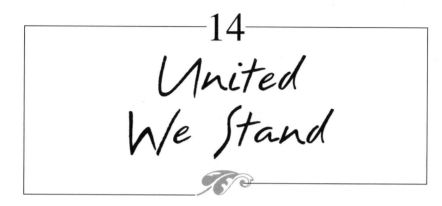

14
United
We Stand

COMBINATIONS OF THERAPIES FOR BEST RESULTS

IN THE preceding chapters we have discussed a number of different factors which may be present in the chain of events leading to rheumatic disease. We have also discussed methods for controlling or treating each factor.

The confounding aspect of rheumatic disease is that these separate factors can go wrong either singly or severally at the same time, and that they can all lead to the same, identical pattern of symptoms from the inflammation produced. Since several things may be simultaneously wrong, you may fully correct one very real problem and still have some symptoms present from the influence of the other antigens. Fortunately, you can use the Daily Total Pain Score to measure step by step the quantitative changes in inflammation that take place as different measures of therapy are undertaken. Occasionally, just one therapy will yield 100 percent relief of pain; but, much more commonly, a combination of measures is needed to achieve substantial relief. All of the therapeutic agents used are relatively natural, and they are compatible with one another.

The first action I take is the establishment of the baseline Total Pain Score. I then select the food elimination diet, or FED, as the first therapeutic step, since it costs nothing, and it is designed to remove antigen. I also routinely recommend vitamin E 800 I.U. daily, vitamin C 1,000 mg daily, beta-carotene 25,000 I.U. daily and EPA (fish oil) about two capsules a day, all helpful in enhancing the defense systems. For patients over the age of 45 I add melatonin 1 to 5 mg at bedtime. After carefully explaining the various therapeutic measures available, I ask patients to make a choice as to what they would like to do next: it's important to take the management of one's own health problem into one's own hands, and patients often have an intuition for what will make them feel better. The exceptions are when an arthritis patient has an additional health problem that can also benefit from a specific one of my arthritis medicines.

For example, when a woman is menopausal or perimenopausal, I will tend to steer her towards female hormonal replacement, because I believe that essentially all menopausal women will enjoy a longer and better quality of life with these medications, regardless of whether they do or do not have rheumatic disease. I feel even more strongly in favor of replacement hormones for diabetic women, because they have a definite increase in uterine cancer, and the progestin hormones will distinctly decrease that cancer potential. The hormones may also slow down the diabetic tendency for arteriosclerosis. If these hormones should help the arthritis, so much the better.

When the patient has hypertension or a history of heart problems, I will steer towards spironolactone, because I believe that this agent is more effective, safer and less expensive than many conventional therapies. If the patient has gout, I will again steer towards spironolactone for its beneficial effect upon the uric acid as well as the accompanying immune complex disease. Most other diuretics tend to accentuate gout.

If a patient should display a nerve type of disturbance, such as a burning pain, numbness or anesthesia, or weakness and paralysis, I start thinking about the benefits of using vitamin B12 plus B1 therapy.

Prednisone, which I commonly use with excellent results, is near the bottom of my sequential list, because its use is often obviated by the therapies that precede it, thereby making the learning of prednisone manipulation a wasted effort. If continuous prednisone is already being used, I usually try decreasing the pain score first with an antigen therapy before recommending the slow and painful discontinuance of the prednisone.

In sum, I tend to use the ideal, antigen-controlling agents first, yet I leave tetracycline until last. This is because tetracycline therapy takes a minimum of four months and may be extended to several years, and many patients are desperately in need of the quick pain "fix" which the other shorter therapies may yield.

More important than the order in which you approach the various therapies is commitment. You must be willing to keep trying the various methods until you have achieved satisfactory pain control and function. And you must resist the feeling of discouragement, which can undermine the best efforts. I suggest that you engage in meditative imagery for its benefits to your arthritis and to your equanimity.

Here to show you how to deduce the value of each therapy through the total pain score are several case reports from my practice. As always, I comment on the interesting lessons to be learned from each person's responses.

When Jessie W #34, briefly mentioned in Chapter 8, first came to see me, she was 46 years old. She told me that she had come down with rheumatic fever at the age of 13, after which she slowly developed many joint pains that were eventually diagnosed as rheumatoid arthritis. When Jessie was in her fortieth year, her condition worsened. She began to suffer intense itching of her arms. (Invisible skin itching is a common manifestation of arthritis.)

She also developed a painful lump under one foot. Her doctor changed the diagnosis to lupus on the basis of a blood test, and started her on daily prednisone. Increasing doses of prednisone on up to 20 mg daily evoked only temporary pain relief, and she began to have trouble walking because of the lump on her foot. Jessie's doctor told her she would eventually need foot surgery. For her serious depression, her doctor added the antidepressant Prozac to her stew of medications.

I determined that Jessie's baseline total pain score was 82. I prescribed spironolactone 100 mg daily, but she could not tolerate it because of nausea. When she proceeded through the FED she found that she was reactive to milk products, pork, crab and watermelon.

By eliminating these, she brought her score down to 50. I next prescribed a tablet containing estrogen and a progestin, but this, too, she did not tolerate. When we tried progestin alone, though, she had no negative reaction and her score came down to 16. At this point I was able to reintroduce spironolactone together with an antinausea medicine and she did fine, and I was soon able to withdraw the antinausea agent. Her scores continued to drop slowly. Feeling much, much better, Jessie also found that she could free herself completely of her antidepressant Prozac. As for the painful nodule under her foot, that disappeared following a regimen of vitamin B12 shots. Coincidentally, the B12 also relieved her intense itching and gave her additional pain relief. Her pain score came down to a very bearable 4. During all this time, Jessie slowly got rid of all her daily prednisone. Jessie now resorts to Microdose prednisone only to relieve occasional slight flares of pain, and averages less than 1 mg prednisone daily.

Jessie's case demonstrates well the synergy that takes place when diet, progestin, spironolactone, Microdose prednisone and vitamin B12 are all marshaled in an attempt to control an arthritis condition. With them, Jessie was relieved of more then 95 percent of her original lupus pain. It might now be appropriate to administer tetracycline to relieve any last bits of pain.

The disappearance of the painful nodule under Jessie's foot happened when the underlying inflammatory disease was brought under control. Accordingly, I delay any consideration of surgical repairs until several months have passed and we have given nature a chance to correct the problem on its own. I look upon surgery—a stressful event—as having the potential to accentuate immune reactivity in patients with rheumatic disease.

Please note that Jessie came to me having taken large amounts of Prozac for several years for depression. During the course of my natural therapies, she came to realize that her depression was lifting; and, with no instruction from me, she reduced her medication in stages until she was taking none. What causes the depression of rheumatic disease? It could be the result of a deficiency of hypothalamic function or CRF (cortisol releasing factor, if you've lost track). But I also believe, from my own experience with arthritis, that it could be a natural reaction to persistent and devastating pain for which there is no realistic expectation for relief.

Jessie also reduced her prednisone essentially to zero, step by step over three months, through paying attention to what her body would tolerate. My role in this was to help her understand why the conventional wisdom of treating lupus with constant, daily suppressive doses of prednisone tends to undermine the body's natural defenses, and then to give her some ideas on how to break free of it. She did the rest. Frankly, I think that the practice of prescribing prednisone is responsible, at least in part, for the poor prognosis for lupus patients generally, and that such a practice is contraindicated for any and all other forms of rheumatic disease as well. Gina P #33, Chapter 8, is a case in point.

Lydia O #46 demonstrates once again how a doctor and patient working together can deduce the right combinations of therapies for the individual. Lydia was 44 when she first came to see me. She was desperate for relief, so much so that she had had her parents drive her 350 miles from home to seek my help. Lydia had experienced the onset of rheumatoid arthritis three years previously. Her problems had begun shortly after her 41st birthday when she had stopped taking birth control pills. Symptoms at first suggested that she was entering early menopause and, coincident with her periods stopping, she experienced hot flashes at night.

She started having pains in many of her joints, and these continued to increase until she could barely function at her workplace or take care of herself at home even with the help of her parents. Any clothing that exerted pressure on Lydia's skin, such as elastics and belts, caused her intolerable pain and swelling. Her local professor rheumatologist had prescribed the usual NSAIDs and, when these proved ineffective, he stepped up treatment by using methotrexate, a powerful cytotoxic drug with many unpleasant side effects, but still she obtained no relief from pain or swelling. Lydia wanted her rheumatologist to let her resume her birth control pills, thinking that there might be a connection between the onset of her pains and the fact that she had stopped taking the hormones, but year after year he would hear none of it. He told her to prepare for a wheelchair in the very near future.

After her mother and father half-carried her into my office, Lydia and I began our doctor-patient relationship with an assessment of her pain. An astonishing baseline total pain score of 231, with almost every joint registering pain and swelling, verified her virtual incapacitation.

My prescription for a birth control pill rapidly brought the total pain score down to 108. The FED produced no change at all. Upon prednisone induction, the total pain score dropped further to 35; but, when Lydia tried to wear restrictive clothing, her score rose again to 72. We next added spironolactone 100 mg daily, and that sent her score tumbling down to 2. Unfortunately the score would would go back up to 17 each month when she stopped the cyclic pill for the week of menstruation. For the seven-day interval I prescribed Microdose prednisone, and that kept her pain score from going up. The combination worked beautifully with 99-plus percent improvement. I last heard from Lydia when she called one day to thank me again. She said she was still following the regimen, and that she was leading an active life once again. As a matter of fact, she was leaving that very day to go deer hunting!

Lydia's remarkable recovery from the brink of helplessness to normal mobility can be attributed to no one agent, but to a combination of progestin, spironolactone and prednisone, as can be seen by the progressive drop in her daily total pain scores. Even though the FED ultimately contributed no improvement in her symptoms, it was important to rule out the role of food as a consideration in designing her therapy. The repeated refusal of her rheumatologist to prescribe her requested hormones afforded me a special opportunity to become a hero and to share her joy when hormones did indeed bring her relief. It is interesting to note, too, that her rheumatologist remained unconvinced that my methods had value, despite the examples of Lydia and several other of his patients with whom I worked with similar favorable results. That doctor joined a cabal to remove my medical license for practicing deceptive medicine!

Lydia and Jessie are also instructive cases in that they provide examples of patients with skin sensitivities. For Lydia it was clothing pressure that produced pain, and for Jessie it was spontaneous itching. In each case the symptom represents irritation of nerve endings in the skin. But the therapies needed proved to be different—spironolactone for Lydia and shots of B12 for Jessie.

B12 also turned out to be the critical element in relieving psoriatic skin lesions in several other cases. Let me relate the stories of Lars and Garson as vivid illustrations.

I first saw farmer Lars A #47 when he was 57 and had suffered from arthritis symptoms for ten years. His troubles started with the diagnosis of gout in his painful right big toe; it was successfully treated with allopurinol. One year later he developed psoriasis all over his body, for which various topical medications provided only minimal relief. Many joint pains started four years after the psoriasis. His doctor tried NSAIDs, methotrexate and sulfasalazine, but achieved no major breakthroughs, though the methotrexate did have a modifying effect on his psoriasis.

Lars, on his own, became aware that he was reactive to citrus fruits and tomatoes, as evidenced by a distinct increase in his arthritis pains shortly after eating them. In particular, his neck became almost immobilized for several days following the ingestion of either of these foods.

Working with me, Lars placed his baseline total pain score at 56. Prednisone induction brought the pain score down to 47. The FED produced no further improvement, though he continued to avoid the citrus fruit and tomatoes as reactive foods. We then tried spironolactone and his score dropped to 30 within the first month and to 20 by the end of the second month. I suggested that he discontinue the methotrexate because of its potentially severe toxicity. However, without the methotrexate, the psoriasis markedly increased in area as well as its redness, roughness, scaling and irritation—to the point where it was becoming more of a problem than his arthritis pain. I put him on vitamin B12 shots weekly. In successive weeks the psoriatic irritation decreased by 50 percent, 60 percent, 65 percent and 75 percent while the redness, roughness and scaling also diminished markedly. Within three months of starting the B12, we both judged the psoriasis to be 80 percent better, as his total pain scores were down to a mere 12. His neck mobility had improved mildly. Lars determined the optimum frequency of the B12 shots to be once every two weeks, and he took over the job of administering them to himself.

Lars's case was ultimately managed through a combination of allopurinol, prednisone, spironolactone, dietary control and vitamin B12. It affected an 80 percent reduction of both his arthritis pain and his psoriatic lesions. Though each additional therapy in itself made only small inroads into Lars's conditions, he would be the first to say that any reduction in discomfort was important to the restoration of a normal life.

There is no information in the medical literature about B12 being involved either in the production of or in the treatment for psoriasis. The exact cause of psoriasis is not known, though it does have an association with immune reactivity along with what is believed to be an inherited basic metabolic abnormality in all the skin tissues, whether they display a psoriatic lesion or not.

The skin cells of a patch of psoriasis reproduce themselves ten times faster than normal. Even the normal skin of a psoriatic person contains twice the normal amount of inflammatory-type chemicals. Methotrexate, an anticancer drug, has been found to be very beneficial in dealing with the lesions of psoriasis. Methotrexate slows down the rapid reproduction of cells by interfering with the production of DNA for cellular reproduction. This inhibitory action is greater in the more rapidly growing cells of psoriasis than in normal cells.

However, methotrexate is also a potent drug the use of which carries the risks of anemia, increased susceptibility to infection, abnormal bleeding and increased cancers.

Vitamin B12, in the production of the genetic DNA material of cells, focuses its action at exactly the same hydrofolate metabolic site as methotrexate. The B12 enhances the normal metabolic process while the methotrexate slows the normal process, yet both have a favorable effect upon the psoriasis. I have no firm answer to that paradox, though I have pointed out a similar paradox in Chapter 5 for vitamin D-calciferol, which both slows down excessive growth of psoriasis and speeds up skin growth for wound healing. I believe that vitamins B12, E and D normalize metabolism. They also assist in the phagocytosis necessary to destroy immune complexes that may theoretically stimulate the rapid skin cellular reproduction. There may still be other normal influences of B12 upon psoriasis that we do not as yet comprehend, such as a possible effect on neuronal activity. Whatever the mechanism may be, the beneficial influence of natural B12 upon psoriasis, as well as upon pain reduction in arthritis, is achieved with immeasurably greater safety and with notably more effectiveness than are the improvements rendered through the use of the artificial, dangerous antimetabolite methotrexate.

The experiences of Garson B #48 parallel those of Lars. Garson was 41 years old when he came to see me about his distressing psoriatic arthritis—arthritis associated with psoriasis. Garson's condition had begun five years earlier when he was 36. Beginning in his fingers and wrists, the arthritis had spread to most of his joints. NSAIDs and gold salts had provided limited pain control and some bad reactions. He showed me a patch of psoriasis the size of a silver dollar on the top of his shiny bald pate; it looked distinctly reddened, raised, scaly and irritated. He reported to me that he was not only physically uncomfortable from this irritating psoriatic lesion, but he was also emotionally distressed by its appearance, which he felt was hampering his career as a salesman. No medications had any significant beneficial influence upon either the psoriasis or the arthritis pain, and though wearing a hair piece to cover the patch made him less self-conscious, he was hoping I could do more for him.

We began with the usual pain tabulation and recorded a baseline total pain score of 76. Prednisone induction brought his total pain score down to 20, but Garson's patch of psoriasis remained unchanged. The FED provided no benefit. After a couple of months, I showed him how to give himself shots of B12—a good idea, as his home was more than 400 miles away. One shot every two weeks brought Garson's pain score down to 5, along with a reduced use of prednisone. The psoriatic lesion stayed about the same size, but the redness faded to a nearly normal color as it became less scaly and peeling. After another month we could see clear signs that normal skin was starting to grow over about 90 percent of the area.

Like the other patients cited above, Garson had found the road to recovery through a process of elimination, and in his case it turned out to be prednisone and vitamin B12. Also, Garson found that the B12 was relevant to both his arthritis and his psoriasis.

Teri C #49 was 69 years old when she consulted me. Her rheumatoid arthritis, which started four years previously, had responded only mildly to Plaquenil, trilisate and intermittent prednisone. She had been taking desensitizing drops under her tongue for milk and wheat allergies detected by RAST testing. She could barely move around because of arthritis pain and stiffness.

Teri's baseline total pain score was 115. When she was placed on the FED and the desensitizing drops were stopped, the score went down to 65 in two weeks, and on down to 20 in six weeks. Chocolate, tomatoes, wheat and caffeine were found to be the reactive foods. For another month the score stayed at about 17. One week after spironolactone 100 mg daily was started, the score was down to 8, and in six weeks it was down to 4. Premarin and Provera were then started as a measure of menopausal maintenance, and the score dropped down to 1 and stayed there. All her previous medications, along with the prednisone and the desensitizing drops, were discontinued completely.

Food, spironolactone and hormones each contributed to this success story. Keep trying until there is little or no pain!

For Teri, the RAST testing missed several reactive foods and incriminated one food, milk, that was not reactive. Stopping the drops (which contain antigen) and getting rid of the reactive foods dropped her pain score 98 points. Her previously expensive food management now costs her nothing. I suspect that a clean deck of tarot cards would have done better than the RAST! Patients Jennifer W #7 and Dierdra L #23 also demonstrate the value of stopping desensitization and removing reactive foods when dealing with arthritis.

Mary C #50 was 69 years old when she brought her three-year-old arthritis problem to me. The onset of the arthritis was sudden and all over her body. NSAIDs helped minimally. Prednisone helped a little, but not enough. Cortisone injections in her knees afforded only temporary relief.

Mary's baseline total pain score was determined to be 87. A prednisone induction dropped the score down to 9. The FED brought the score down to 4. Spironolactone now has the score between zero and 1. Microdose prednisone controls rare, small flares, with the dosage averaging less than 1 mg per day.

Prednisone, FED and spironolactone each had a hand in producing good results. The original major importance of prednisone was diminished, but not eliminated, by the agents controlling antigen.

You may have noticed in the case histories cited in this chapter that tetracycline for bacteria was not used. At the time these patients were in my care, the use of antibiotics for arthritis was in its infancy, and I lacked exact prescribing details. I believe rheumatic therapy is not complete until all three antigen factors—food, hormones and bacteria—have been addressed or the pain score has gone to zero. As I look back on these cases, I could wish that I had added tetracycline to the sequence of therapies tried. Prednisone figured prominently in some cases. As you know from reading this book, I prefer to control symptoms through the elimination of antigen as much as possible in the belief that by diminishing the antigen reaction I can help to reduce the long-term sensitization and reactivity. As Burnet (1967) said long ago, the ideal therapy for immune disease is to remove the antigen. After that ideal principle has been fully applied and some symptoms should still remain, I then think that prednisone given by Microdose would become the *pièce de résistance!* The use of glucosamine would also be appropriate at this time.

In summary, anyone with rheumatic disease must keep in mind that the most effective management of this complex, multisymptomed disorder must be achieved through a combination of therapeutic measures. Each measure, on the average, provides only a limited percentage of the total success in treatment. Speaking with many years of experience in treating many hundreds of cases, I can say that progestins help about 50 percent of patients, spironolactone about 50 percent, antibiotics about 50 percent, B12 about 50 percent, and the elimination of foods another 25-30 percent. In combinations tailored to the individual, they should yield an average of about 90 percent pain relief in patients who use them. It must be stressed again that success comes in steps rather than in one great leap, and that arthritis sufferers must learn patience and be grateful for each successive measure of improvement, be it large or small.

REMEMBER

1. The Daily Total Pain Score is invaluable for its ability to monitor the individual values of each successive arthritis therapy.
2. Your rheumatic disease may be due to a combination of causative factors.
3. Different therapies, although introduced in any sequence one at a time, may ultimately be used simultaneously once their value has been established.
4. The Food Elimination Diet is attractive as your first investigative measure because it costs nothing and has no negative side effects.
5. Give priority to arthritis medications the patient should take for other existing health reasons.
6. Unless infection is clearly implicated at the start, it is preferable to leave antibiotic therapy until last, because it can take so long to get results.
7. Vitamin B12 may help skin itchiness, pain and psoriasis. B12 supersedes methotrexate in safety, cost and effectiveness for treating both arthritis pain and psoriasis.
8. The standard treatment of lupus with constant prednisone may explain at least in part why the prognosis for lupus is so poor.

15
Manipulating The Immune System

ARE NSAIDS APPROPRIATE?

UNQUESTIONABLY, THE ideal therapy for rheumatic disease is the removal of the causative antigen, whatever its origin. However, when an obscure antigen cannot be identified or removed, and very severe symptoms persist, the only practical course of action is to try to reduce the pain of the disease process. One method of treating this type of resistant problem is to influence the patient's immune system. The question is, influence it in what direction? Is it better to enhance the function of the immune system or to depress it?

The answer starts with looking at how the immune system works. The immune system first produces antibodies that can neutralize an antigen invader by forming an antibody-antigen immune complex, and then provides macrophages that digest and rid the blood of that immune complex.

When more immune complexes are made than can be destroyed,

the excess complexes filter out into the tissues to produce the inflammation of rheumatic disease. To counter that unfavorable balance, two therapeutic strategies are available. The first is to reduce or depress the natural production of antibody so that there will be fewer immune complexes formed. The second is to improve the function of the phagocytes so that more immune complexes can be destroyed. The consensus of modern medical authorities is that the former is the more effective strategy in controlling rheumatic disease. Accordingly, much attention has been given to systems of medication that depress immune function, chiefly with a group of drugs classified as immunosuppressants.

Methotrexate, which is chiefly an anticancer drug, has also been a favorite immunosuppressive agent used to treat rheumatoid arthritis when simpler treatments have proved ineffective. Methotrexate has toxic, potentially dangerous effects on the liver, lungs and red blood cells. It increases susceptibility to certain cancers and to serious infections. It can produce intestinal bleeding and perforation. Its therapeutic impact isn't significant until you have been on it for two or three months, and its effectiveness frequently diminishes after two or three years. People taking it for severe rheumatoid arthritis average about 23 percent reduction of pain. The therapeutic purpose of methotrexate is to slow down lymphocyte reproduction and antibody production. The fact that it also slows down vital phagocytic activity seems to have escaped serious medical attention.

The substantial adverse effects, including blood disorders, attributable to immunosuppressive agents have limited their use in rheumatic diseases. Irradiation of lymphatic portions of the body and the use of serum containing antibodies which destroy T-cells also have detriments which far outweigh their benefits.

Emotional stress is increasingly recognized as a depressor of immune function. It is also well known that stress rapidly accentuates the symptoms of rheumatic disease, and that prolonged stress increases the incidence of cancer and earlier-than-expected death.

One of the consequences of emotional stress is believed to be the depression of the function of the lymphocytes and the consequent reduction of the number of immune complexes formed. This is very similar to the effect that immunodepressive therapeutic agents have on the production of immune complexes. But in real life we find that emotional stress actually increases the symptoms of arthritis rather than decreasing them. I propose that emotional stress in all likelihood depresses the function of the macrophages more than it does that of the lymphocytes; this is one theory that makes sense of this effect of stress on arthritis. Though I search the literature constantly, I am not aware of such macrophage function being measured in rheumatic disease in the laboratory as yet. However, we must consider another possible explanation. Stress may decrease the amount of active serotonin, which can lead to a decreased function of the hypothalamus, which in turn can lead to decreased cortisol surges. The result in this scenario, too, is increased rheumatic pain.

The enzymatic enhancement of folate metabolism by vitamin B12 is exactly opposed to the inhibition of folate metabolism by methotrexate. In a group of 36 rheumatic patients treated with B12 injections, I found a 33 percent pain improvement overall. In contrast, the pain control benefit recorded in a seven-year study of patients treated with methotrexate was about 23 percent overall, a significant difference. Another contrasting factor to be taken into account is safety. B12 has essentially no dangerous reactions associated with its use. B12 is also more effective for the control of psoriasis than methotrexate, as demonstrated in Chapter 14. And B12 is immensely less expensive. The cost of just your first of many regular visits to the doctor and laboratory for methotrexate therapy far exceeds the annual cost for B12 self-administration at home (less than $50 per year at most).

Looking at those comparisons, one might wonder why methotrexate is ever used. Sadly, when everything else has failed and the intensity of pain constantly interferes with their functioning and sleep, many patients are driven to risk the possible lethal effects of methotrexate in order to reduce their intolerable pain. It is also true that B12's value is still not recognized in the medical profession; thus, methotrexate therapy has been the patient's only option. One reason that the medical profession does not yet know about B12 and my other therapies is that they close their eyes, ears, minds and their doors when I have tried to approach them, now over the course of many years while I have been making the patients they failed with better!

Modern therapy for emotional stress and depression is typically managed with quick-fix tranquilizers and other antianxiety drugs. But these expensive drugs do not address the source of the stress and depression. Better by far is to learn through reading, tapes, counseling and group therapy how to manage your life in such a way as to either avoid the factors causing stress or find better ways to accommodate to them. Caffeine is stressful, depressive and causative of arthritis, but were you ever advised to not drink caffeine as your tranquilizer prescription was being written? My patients got advice.

WHERE DO IMMUNE COMPLEXES COME FROM?

The theory espoused by the majority of modern rheumatologists is that there are two sources of immune complexes that produce joint inflammation: one portion is formed in the joint by mobile, joint-specific antibodies which combine with immobile joint tissue antigens (autoimmune disease); and a second portion is formed by mobile antibodies which combine with mobile antigens circulating throughout the body. According to this theory, the immobile joint complexes join in with the circulating complexes that filter into the joint to collaborate in the process of joint inflammation.

My own view is significantly different. I propose that the entire supply of immune complexes is made by the union of specific mobile antibodies with their specific mobile antigens at sites remote from the joints. If, as happens in rheumatic disease, they are not consumed by phagocytes, they are free to enter the joints, where they create inflammation. The autoimmune aspect of arthritis is enacted by specific antibodies joining with mobile steroid hormone antigenic complexes (homemade or autoimmune), which travel to the joint with other immune complexes to create inflammation. I strongly doubt that disease-producing antibodies attach themselves to joint tissues. I present the following three basic observations as evidence in support of my theory.

Observation #1: Sometimes when I remove a reactive food from a patient's diet, rheumatic symptoms are relieved 100 percent. At times when spironolactone or tetracycline are administered, symptoms are 100 percent relieved. Sometimes combinations of the above three are necessary to achieve full relief. None of these therapeutic measures has any relevance to the production of anti-joint antibodies or the union of antibodies and joint tissue antigens. If even a fraction of the symptoms of these same patients were due to joint-specific antibodies, then the relief for these patients could not be 100 percent.

Observation #2: A basic element of my therapy for every single rheumatic patient is to enhance the function of the immune system through supplementation with specific vitamins (see Chapter 5). In the majority of cases, total pain scores have been improved by vitamins alone; the minority of patients notice no difference; I have never detected even a slight worsening of joint pain as a result of these vitamin supplements, as conventional theories might predict. This causes me to conclude that there has been no symptomatic, direct antibody-joint tissue antigen reaction in any of the hundreds of patients I have treated. I therefore doubt that such a local, disease-producing, tissue-antibody reaction occurs at all; and, if it does exist, that it is responsible for only an imperceptible, negligible percentage of the total disease. All antibodies do not produce disease, as exemplified by ''diagnostic'' rheumatoid arthritis antibodies being found in perfectly healthy people.

Observation #3: Some patients experience arthritis pains only periodically, as in gout or palindromic arthritis; likewise, some patients experience periods of spontaneous remission. Given that immunity is a sensitization that lasts throughout the life of the individual, particularly when joint antigen is constantly present to stimulate and boost that immunity, it seems unrealistic to consider that arthritis based on that specific antibody-joint target tissue reaction could come and go periodically. On the other hand, it is very reasonable to think that an immune response based on a reactive food could produce arthritic pains only in response to ingesting that food, and that progesterone allergy can cause arthritis pains only at the time when reactive progesterone is produced in the menstrual cycle. In the intervening times of no antigen, the joint is silent.

There are important implications for therapy in the distinctly different theories underlying the cause of arthritis. If we are to believe the old theory, the joints can only become more reactive to disease as time goes on. Since it would not be possible to remove all painful joint and organ antigen involved in rheumatic disease, depression of the immune system would become a reasonable therapy for relieving pain. If, however, we accept my new theory as a reasonable approach, then it becomes logical to focus efforts on first, removing all sources of antigen and, second, on enhancing the function of the immune system so as to dispose of the arthritis-producing immune complexes before they have a chance to enter joints and destroy joint tissues.

You can readily see in the foregoing analysis that there are two opposite approaches to relieving rheumatic disease: the former based on depressing the immune system and the latter on enhancing it. I look upon *depression of the immune system* as counter to nature. One experiences not only all of the direct adverse effects of using alien therapeutic chemicals, such as NSAIDs and methotrexate, but also the indirect adverse effects of living without the protection inherent in a system of natural defenses that exist to protect us from diseases. It is all too likely that the patient receiving immunosuppressive therapy will end up in worse health than if he or she had received no therapy at all! Also, while undergoing methotrexate therapy there is no hope for ultimate health, because therapy must continue until death.

By contrast, I look upon *enhancement of the immune system* as consistent with nature's own medicine, with the body's inherent systems for self-healing being enhanced and utilized to their maximum. In boosting the immune system, one uses only normal, natural therapeutic agents that have neither direct nor indirect adverse effects. It is virtually impossible for these agents to put you into worse health after treatment. In view of all this, the logical, healthy choice seems obvious.

There are some autoimmune diseases in which antibody combines directly with tissue antigen, and that concerns red blood cells for immune hemolytic anemia, and platelets for immune thrombocytopenia. Immunosuppression is apparently of distinct value in this type of case. I do not want you to think that immunosuppression should be totally discarded; it may be the only way to improve the quality of life for those patients for whom nothing else is working and rheumatic pain is severe. My goal at this time is to convince rheumatologists to try my new and better/safer/cheaper system as the starting point on their therapeutic program in the expectation that it will work and work well.

NSAIDs, Are They Friends or Foes?

I have been making the case that use of the immunosuppressive drugs of modern rheumatological therapy has little justification other than in the extreme cases where nothing else has helped to relieve severe pain. Similarly, I believe that nonsteroidal anti-inflammatory drugs should be limited to those cases in which all other reasonable therapy has failed.

NSAID, remember, is the acronym for Nonsteroidal Anti-Inflammatory Drug. NSAIDs are so called and so advertised because they avoid the use of steroids, such as cortisone, which were previously considered to be extremely dangerous; but now, as you know, the correct use of the steroids according to the Microdose system makes steroids a very helpful and entirely safe ally in arthritis therapy.

The first recognized NSAID was aspirin, acetylsalicylic acid, which came into use for arthritis pain at the end of the 19th century and gave mild relief for some arthritis pain, up to about 20 percent. The principal problem with aspirin was that it had entirely too many side effects, including stomach ulceration and hemorrhage, ringing in the ears, changes in vision, liver disturbances and even kidney damage when used in persistently high doses associated with chronic arthritis treatment. Because of these problems, our pharmaceutical industry has been developing other aspirinlike drugs that might relieve the pain at least as well as aspirin does, but without the same severe side effects. Alternative NSAID products now exist that have partly diminished the degree of stomach ulceration, though they are far from completely safe. Stomach hemorrhage, stomach perforation and kidney damage remain a serious concern, while other difficulties have appeared or increased with these aspirin substitutes, including vision, liver and blood damage. Rashes, allergies and emotional changes also trouble some users.

The NSAIDs are effective because they diminish inflammation

and pain by blocking the production of prostaglandins, the chemicals that cause inflammation and trigger transmission of pain signals to the brain. (See Figure 5-1, page 69.) Pain and swelling are ordinarily protective measures that make you aware of an injury so that you will protect it sufficiently to allow it time to heal. The problem in arthritis is that the site of inflammation fails to heal completely, so that the pain and inflammation become chronic.

Arthritis sufferers who depend upon NSAIDs for long-term relief of pain tend to end up having overused them. James Fries, M.D., estimates that the number of people who die each year in the U.S.A. from the use of NSAIDs may be as high as 20,000, and that there are well over 100,000 hospitalizations annually due to NSAIDs. About 15 percent—roughly 20,000—of ongoing renal dialysis cases are the result of excess NSAID medication over a long period of time.

Consequently, my advice to arthritis sufferers is to carefully avoid NSAIDs. I do not prescribe or recommend them, because I want a trouble-free life with trouble-free patients. I must add, however, that there may be times when your own judgment says that your immediate pain is great enough to outweigh the relatively small danger from *temporary* use of the over-the-counter NSAIDs. I do suggest the use of occasional acetaminophen (Tylenol) for mild pain relief, because it is kinder to the stomach, but Tylenol is still tougher on the kidneys than aspirin in the long run.

Many NSAID alternatives to aspirin have been developed to decrease the stomach acid problem, and they all claim to be the very best at it, but they are all pretty much the same. A 25-mg tablet is no better than a 600-mg dose—such claims are sales gimmicks. Every manufacturer of NSAIDs has given the required honest report in *Physicians' Desk Reference* that their product is associated with fatalities from intestinal hemorrhage, stomach perforation, kidney disease and liver inflammation. These replacement drugs may also, among many other reported problems, have an adverse influence upon hearing, vision, asthma and anemia. A more or less complete list of products classified as NSAIDs includes Advil, Aleve, Anaprox, Ansaid, Clinoril, Dolobid, Feldene, Indocin, Lodine, Meclomen, Motrin, Nalfon, Naprosyn, Orudis, Oruvail, Ponstel, Relafen, Tolectin, Toradol and Voltaren.

NSAIDs are directed at inhibiting inflammatory products after the basic immune complex reaction has occurred, but they do not stop the immune reaction. The NSAIDs do a cover-up job while the main disease progresses. I believe that when NSAIDs are advertised as allowing you to go jogging today, they are jeopardizing your healthy tomorrow by coaxing you to further damage your already unhealthy cartilage. My antigen treatments are aimed at stopping that immune reaction from ever occurring. To make an exaggerated comparison, I remove the atomic bomb rather than trying to clear up the radiation effects after it has exploded.

When taking your NSAIDs regularly, you might have to make periodic visits to the laboratory for liver and blood tests, to your eye doctor for vision tests, to your stomach doctor for ulcer evaluations, to your surgeon for ulcer repair or removal, and to your heart doctor for fluid collection and kidney backup. The people who are most likely to get into a kidney problem with NSAIDs are those who are taking diuretics, have heart failure, have liver malfunction, have kidney malfunction and are elderly. A large study of patients on NSAIDs reported that 9.4 percent dropped out because they could not tolerate adverse reactions, 15 percent of patients had an elevated liver enzyme reaction, and 17 percent of patients had a hemoglobin drop of 1 gm or more from internal bleeding or interference with normal blood replacement.

When the combination of NSAIDs' dangerous side effects and the limited reduction of pain is weighed against the positive results of antigen removal and immune system enhancement, the choice seems to speak for itself. In my view, the only justification for using NSAIDs is failure to respond to any other methods of treatment, and my guess is that only a fraction of one percent of patients fall into that category. In my own fifteen years of working with patients with rheumatoid diseases, I have only rarely found anyone who could not be made better without them.

GLUCOSAMINE VERSUS NSAIDs

Some researchers find that NSAIDs degrade joint cartilage, while others find that some do and some don't. In general, NSAIDs put the joint cartilage at risk, while it is agreed that glucosamine tends to protect or reestablish cartilage health. Pain is a natural protection which immobilizes damaged joints so that the cartilage will not be further destroyed by the rubbing from physical activity. NSAIDs, which tend to further diminish the integrity of the joint cartilage by their biochemical activity, also tend to relieve the protective joint pain so that uninhibited physical activity can further damage the joint tissues—a case of double damage.

NSAIDs have been found to relieve rheumatic pain more quickly than glucosamine at first, but at four weeks they are equal, and at eight weeks the glucosamine produces slightly greater relief. We can also consider the observation that NSAIDs provide diminishing pain control over the course of several months, while the improvements of glucosamine are reported to be maintained unabated not only as long as the medication is continued, but for one to three months after it is stopped. In my opinion, NSAIDs are entirely too lethally dangerous for chronic arthritis therapy, they slowly lose their pain control, and they do not help heal the damaged joint cartilage. Glucosamine has a reasonable potential for both pain relief and cartilage healing without any known dangers.

Why isn't this product used more in the U.S.A.? Pharmaceutical companies cannot patent it to make millions of dollars in profit, so they are unwilling to spend the millions necessary to prove its efficacy beyond a reasonable doubt, and unwilling to spend large sums advertising. Therefore, glucosamine remains quietly on the shelves of your natural food stores hoping you will find it and use it. I knew essentially nothing about it until I read *The Arthritis Cure*, because most rheumatology texts do not even mention its name.

REMEMBER

1. Therapeutic depression of the immune system may lead to more serious problems than it controls—cancer, infection and death.
2. Problem-free vitamin enhancement (B12) of the immune system is far more effective in inflammation and pain control than methotrexate suppression.
3. My clinical evidence indicates that there is no demonstrable symp-

tomatic antibody attachment to joint tissues, and this fact puts into question the logic of methotrexate immunosuppression.

4. NSAIDs have provided only limited relief of arthritis pain, and chronic use puts the individual at risk for stomach and kidney damage.

5. Logical, safe and effective rheumatic control is through antigen removal and immune system enhancement.

6. Glucosamine has no adverse effects and it has pain-relieving powers about equal to aspirin's after a few weeks.

7. Glucosamine reportedly helps heal cartilage.

—16—

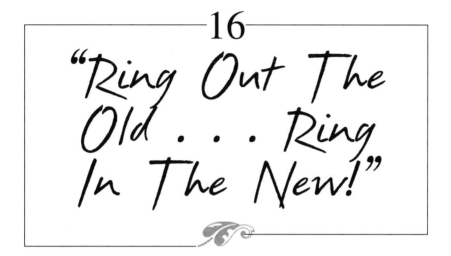
"Ring Out The Old . . . Ring In The New!"

THE NSAIDS CAUSE THE RINGING!

I BELIEVE that this book has amalgamated a hodgepodge of standard arthritis information into a rational and very meaningful system of understanding. This new system is immeasurably more effective, safer and less costly than standard rheumatological therapy. I expect that by reading, learning and understanding this information, you will have gained what amounts to a nearly medical level of knowledge about rheumatic disease. I trust that what you have learned will be of greater assistance in attaining better health and comfort than you had previously believed possible. There is a very realistic hope for your recovery from arthritis. I dearly hope that, if and when you should find it necessary to engage the services of a physician to prescribe your medicines, you will be able to teach him the principles you have learned, not only for your benefit, but also for the benefit of his other patients as well. If you buy an extra copy of this book for your doctor, it will be a small but worthwhile investment in your therapeutic success.

I expect that this book will serve as a reference for you from time to time, and that you will read it more than once, since there are so many facts to learn and several points of logic to mull over. What you learn towards the end of the book will put more meaning into what you have read at the beginning of the book, so the second reading will be still more informative.

It is my hope that among the many patients whose case reports have been presented you have found at least one with whom you can personally identify so that you have a better inner feeling for the realistic possibilities for your own rheumatic improvement.

REVIEW OF THE BASIC ETIOLOGY OF RHEUMATIC DISEASE

All forms and names of arthritis represent the one and only basic disease of excess immune complex irritation/inflammation with the pattern of rheumatic disease determined genetically.

The immune system consists of your lymphocytes and your phagocytes. The lymphocytes function to make antibody against alien antigens. Circulating antibody combines with circulating antigen to form immune complexes. There is little to no evidence that pathogenic antibodies attach themselves to immobile joint tissue or organ tissue antigens in rheumatic disease. The phagocytes' function is to digest immune complexes and thereby form the primary defense against immune inflammation. The lymphocytes and phagocytes coordinate to intercept and destroy all factors perceived as alien.

You have learned that cortisol acts as an anti-inflammatory agent in very large pulses from the adrenals in response to hypothalamic cortisol releasing factor (CRF), and thereby forms the secondary defense against immune inflammation. (See Figure 2-1, page 21.) Active rheumatic disease is associated with inadequate CRF production by the hypothalamus. Hypothalamic exhaustion from excessive stimulation is usually the result of arthritis inflammation rather than the cause of it. The exhausted hypothalamus can recuperate and then return to normal function after being rested by periodic prednisone supplementation. Hypothalamic unresponsiveness produced by excessive stimulation is a natural protection against the dangers of continuous, excessive cortisol production. The adrenal glands can also return to normal function, even after many years of constant suppression.

The excess of immune complexes, which overwhelm the immune system's ability to destroy them, filter out of the circulation into the joints and other tissues, where they react with complement to produce inflammatory products. Inflammation begins when the cortisol defensive system is unable to inactivate all of the inflammatory products. The event that heralds the onset of lupus in genetically predisposed mice is the loss of phagocytic power to ingest immune complexes.

The maximal production of immune complexes is normally determined by the size of the antigen supply rather than by the antibody supply. The normal supply of immune complexes is greatly increased in number by three main groups of "alien" antigen—foods, hormones and microbes, and by any combination of these three agents. Though the antigens are chemically different from one another, they are semi-equalized to one another as they form an immune complex. All three produce the identical pain pattern in any one person with arthritis. The pain intensity is due to the combined sum of whatever immune complexes are present.

Gout is primarily an immune complex rheumatic disease and secondarily a flaw in uric acid metabolism.

Reaction to native hormone is clearly an autoimmune disease, while reaction to foods and microbes is plain immune disease. Therefore, arthritis is a combination of autoimmune and immune disease.

The potential antigenic complexes produced by gynecic tissues can produce autoimmune arthritis as well as a cyclic anesthesia and paralysis syndrome which is similar to multiple sclerosis. (This topic is treated in detail in Appendix A.) The progesterone for forming the potential antigenic complexes can arise either from the ovaries or from the adrenal glands.

Review of Basic Therapy for Rheumatic Disease

The Daily Total Pain Score is always essential to measure the degree of positive influence or lack of influence of each separate therapeutic measure or agent being used. Its sensitivity is equal to or greater than a physician's daily physical examination.

The basic principles of antirheumatic therapy apply to all forms of rheumatic disease regardless of name. The ideal rheumatic therapy is to remove or block the antigenic food/hormone/microbes step by step so that immune reactions do not occur. Reactive foods are detected by the Food Elimination Diet and then removed from your custom-made diet. Hormones are eliminated or blocked by progestins and spironolactone. Mycoplasma microbes are eradicated by antibiotics of the tetracycline group.

Perhaps not ideal, yet very excellent, therapy is to be found in supporting your natural primary and secondary inflammation defense systems. This amounts to enhancement of the immune system rather than depression of the immune system, as would be recommended by rheumatologists.

Your primary inflammation defense of phaging immune complexes may be bolstered by antioxidant vitamin supplements which increase the eating and digestive powers of your phagocytes. This includes vitamin B12 by injection and oral E, C, B1, beta-carotene and EPA. The hormone melatonin acts as an antioxidant as well as a direct stimulator of immune function.

Your secondary inflammation defense may be enhanced by the judicious use of prednisone with the Microdose system. (See Figure 2-1, page 21). Five-day prednisone administration supplants deficient CRF cortisol pulses while it rests the hypothalamus for recuperation. Megadoses of vitamins B12 and B1 improve hypothalamic function through their ability to enhance nerve function.

We are now down to the third level of therapy for control of local tissue inflammation. The antioxidants, particularly E and C, along with EPA, help to control inflammation and unusual blood vessel clotting. Melatonin is particularly effective against DNA oxidation. These agents do not relieve pain as well as the NSAIDs, but they are immeasurably safer and have added values for future good health, such as inhibiting arteriosclerosis.

Vitamin B12 is closely associated with function of the immune system as well as the function of nerves. An elevated immune tissue or nerve tissue threshold to B12 requires frequent megadosage therapy, which at times may be as often as every two days. The B12 must be given by injection in order to attain the required supranormal blood levels.

Spironolactone may remove antigenic steroid hormones either by altering steroidogenesis of the ovaries, testicles and adrenals, and/or it may block steroid hormonal receptor sites.

Spironolactone works synergistically with allopurinol in gouty arthritis to enhance tissue health by control of abnormal uric acid metabolism, and it also may inhibit rheumatic inflammation by control of hormonal antigen.

Psychoneuroimmunology is now being used for arthritis control in some medical centers with the use of the power of positive thinking, hypnosis, self-hypnosis and attacking your disease with your own mind and imagery. A visit to a certified psychologist-hypnotherapist could organize your plans for self management. Daily meditation presents a real possibility for establishing a healthier life with greater equanimity. Healing by touch is also of value.

I recommend estrogen replacement therapy in the menopause for all women, for bone preservation, longevity and a better quality of life, and particularly for those women with arthritis, which adds to bone destruction.

The problems that arise with gynecic autoimmunity can usually be treated with exogenous hormones, but sometimes it becomes necessary to do an extensive surgical reduction of the gynecic tissues to bring a powerful disease under control. (See Appendix A for a full discussion of this.)

There is evidence to indicate that glucosmine sulfate heals joint cartilage, and it also relieves arthritis pain and inflammation about as well as the NSAIDs. There are no known serious adverse reactions. The manner in which glucosamine and its accompanying chondroitin relieve pain has not been determined.

Twenty minutes or more of daily exercise within the limits of joint comfort is very important for maintaining your general health and bone strength.

I discourage the use of NSAIDs, DMARDs and methotrexate because of their frequently lethal complications, huge cost and minimal relief of pain.

There is no one measure of therapy that fixes all arthritis problems. Fixing is a matter of correcting that specific factor or combination of factors which might be wrong. You have seen that a combination of therapies may have an incremental success that adds up to a high percentage of pain control. *E pluribus unum* is the logical motto for my arthritis theory and therapy: diverse medication produce one logical, cohesive and effective regimen.

A diagram of rheumatic disease, Figure 16-1, serves to give you an overview of the natural development of the excess immune complex disease called arthritis.

As I conclude my arthritis message to you, I would like to acknowledge the master herbalists, who are acquainted with the special functions and powers of the countless herbs of our planet—which I most definitely am not. Herbalists have both victories and failures in their attempts to relieve arthritis suffering. I believe their batting average is not as good as mine, but I am still ready to refer my failures to their care. Their occasional ''miracles'' bolster my willingness. I don't care what system is used for improving health and comfort as long as it has a reasonable chance for success and is done without danger to the patient. When we all work as a team, we have the best chance for reaching the ideal.

RING OUT THE OLD . . .

There comes a time in every endeavor when we must stop and consider whether we are really doing the correct thing, particularly when the results are less than desired. The medical treatment of arthritis has been going on for many long years, but the results have not drawn many accolades. I have presented a new and logical theory for arthritis etiology and a very effective system of rheumatic therapy, which together clearly outshine the old systems of theory and therapy. The excellence of pain improvement for some patients now extends up to 100 percent.

. . . RING IN THE NEW!

Please do not be deluded into believing that this book represents the final word in rheumatic immune disease control, but do look at it as a long step forward. I believe that everything I have said in this book

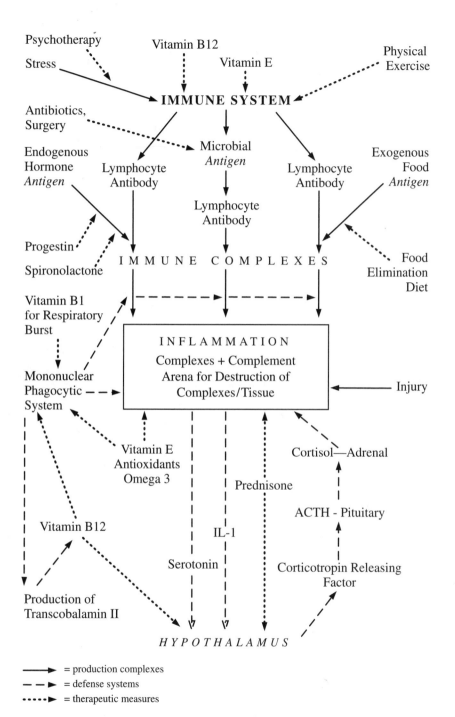

Figure 16-1. United Arthritis Concepts

is right, or I would not have said it. I trust that I have transmitted to you the knowledge and the logic behind the medical beliefs that I hold very firmly, so that you also can believe them strongly enough to courageously pursue relief of your arthritis. However, I do hope that the scientists in the future will have opportunities to add new features; because, each time they do, they will improve upon the successful treatment of this prevalent and devastating disease of arthritis—the ultimate goal for us all.

A COMMITMENT

My concerns and interests do not end with the writing of this book. I am exceedingly interested in the future progress of these concepts about immune disease in the practice of medicine for the benefit of arthritis sufferers. I would like to receive constructive criticisms of my concepts and therapies from patients and physicians alike. Your reports about good results from the therapies I have recommended will be appreciated as well as any unsatisfactory results. I would welcome the opportunity to assist in formulating the plans of research groups. I will arrange for lectures or discussions with interested lay or professional groups. All your written questions by mail will be answered with reasonable promptness. My mailing address is 21 Sarcka Lane, Litchfield, CT 06759. When I am available, I will accept telephone calls—only from physicians—at 860-567-8855, but I do not return calls unless collect. I will be happy to discuss matters, but I do not prescribe at any time, since that must always be done by your doctor.

If there are some of you who would like to contribute financially to further research of that which has helped your arthritis do so much better, I offer to be your agent to see that your support goes completely and directly to an appropriate investigative group of physicians.

Appendix A

GYNECIC TISSUES: THE CYCLIC ANESTHESIA AND PARALYSIS SYNDROME

THE FOLLOWING information about gynecic (ji-nee'-sik) tissues will help you understand the basic concepts about their prominent role in the potential production of arthritis. The tissues of the genital ridge of the embryo are the source of the ovaries, fallopian tubes, uterus, cervix, a cuff of the vagina and the round ligaments. The round ligaments consist mainly of smooth muscle and fibrous connective tissue, and they hold the uterus in place. I have applied the term *gynecic tissues* to all those tissues which grow out from the genital ridge of the embryo. I group them together because of their common origin, and also because I believe that they all have the potential of making an antigenic protein that may bind with a hapten progesterone to form an antigen, or antigenic complex. I believe that such progesterone-protein antigenic complexes, after being united with antibody and then combined with complement at various target tissue sites throughout the body, may cause irritation and inflammation.

Heredity determines the patterns of immune disease which tend to be common in certain family lines. According to the variable target tissue being attacked, even though the basic irritative-inflammatory mechanism is identical, there may be varyingly named diseases: arthritis, dysmenorrhea, PMS, cyclic anesthesia and paralysis syndrome, endometriosis, etc. These are all termed immune diseases and in large part are autoimmune or immune-to-yourself diseases in that the antigenic factors that cause the disease are constructed by the body itself. If a prescription progestin is causing the arthritis, it is not a true autoimmune disease, because the antigen is not made by the body itself, although the basic mechanism of disease production is identical to that of native progesterone.

We have discussed in Chapter 6 that there are different forms of progesterone produced by the ovary and that the progesterones are also produced in varying quantities. We also concluded that our prime concern is the progesterone quality relative to the immune system, rather than the quantity or hormonal balance. I would also like to note now that progesterone is also made by the adrenal glands, as far as we know, on a constant rather than a cyclic basis.

PMS is a commonly used acronym for premenstrual syndrome. A syndrome is a group of associated signs and symptoms. Medically, PMS stands for all the *cyclic* problems that occur in connection with menstruation (more specifically ovulation), and that most commonly include pain, increased bleeding, bloating and emotional tension. To call it premenstrual tension is rather inaccurate, because the entire syndrome may occur at the time of ovulation, premenstrually or intramenstrually, or even at a combination of all three times. Additionally, the identical cyclic syndrome of pain and tension can occur after a simple hysterectomy when there is no vaginal bleeding or menstruation whatsoever, so that in fact it is *not* always associated with menstruation, but with the ovulatory cycle and specifically, with the type of progesterone the ovulating ovary is making at the time.

The symptoms of dysmenorrhea, which include pain and tension, are associated with ovulatory menstruation. Some menses may occur without ovulation, and they probably will be comfortable. Painless and tension-free menstruation can be produced, therefore, by spontaneous anovulation or by ovulation-inhibiting medicines. Oral contraceptives both block ovulation and replace native progesterone with a (hopefully) nonreactive progestin.

I performed an experiment (Irwin et al. 1981) with informed consent in which I withdrew two pints of blood from the arms of several women with severe dysmenorrhea, the first pint at the time of pain and tension, and the second pint at a time of no symptoms. I then did hysterectomies for many of them. A few months after the hysterectomies, the pints of blood were transfused on separate days back into their donors who did not know which pint they were receiving. The pain-associated pints reproduced pain and tension, while the no-pain pints produced nothing. The average time delay between the transfusion and the onset of symptoms was four to five hours, and that timing suggests that the causative factor in the blood was immune-related rather than an immediately toxic chemical, such as a prostaglandin. The average duration of pain produced was about eight hours. These observations strongly suggest that immune complexes circulating in the blood at the time of dysmenorrhea and tension are causative of those symptoms and that the symptoms produced will disappear shortly after the production of complexes has stopped. One of the transfusion recipients called me six hours later to report that: "It was such a beautiful day! I felt perfectly well, and everything was favorable and happy, but now I have started to cry like a baby and I can't stop! I can't figure out why!"

The rules that govern the pattern of progesterone immune complexes affecting dysmenorrhea should be identical to the rules that govern the pattern of progesterone immune complexes affecting arthritis. This is verified by the patients who experience the cyclical occurrence of simultaneous dysmenorrhea and arthritis.

Some of my patients, who had the standard hysterectomy with the tubes and ovaries retained, gradually developed severe cyclic symptoms of pain, fever and emotional irritability which required my reoperating to remove the remaining tubes and ovaries to control the problem. I began to reason: Generally, when the uterus alone is removed the pain problem is removed, but not always. Big pains are made by the uterus, while smaller pains are made by the residual tissues. I then started removing both tubes and one ovary at the time of hysterectomy with improved, but not perfect, control of residual cyclic pain. When I added a cuff of vagina and the round ligaments out to the inguinal ring to my list for surgical removal, the control of residual problems was nearly perfect. The round ligaments cannot be removed completely, because they extend out into the major lips. I have come to believe that, by reducing the residual gynecic tissue mass to below a certain critical threshold level while still retaining one ovary, the production of potential antigenic protein is essentially eliminated. I like to leave one normal, healthy ovary in young women for spontaneous, natural good health; but, if endometriosis or adhesive pelvic disease is present, then I will remove both ovaries as well, because of their potentially bad performance, not only for what I believe is an increased potential for ovarian cancer, but also for the high degree of immune sensitivity of the residual tissues in these inflammatory immune disease manifestations that may persist in spite of the reduced, but not eliminated, gynecic volume.

When one ovary alone is retained upon removing all available gynecic tissue, it continues to ovulate regularly and continues to produce the same hapten progesterone, but there are no residual symptoms. I conclude that this occurs because of limited-to-no production of potential antigenic protein. With the knowledge of this performance, I have been supplied with the courage to approach some rather unusual problems in severely distressed young women in a manner that brings success to my patients, but produces stress in my fellow physicians who have never taken the time or effort to listen and learn about what I do and why I do it.

REMEMBER

1. Gynecic tissue is a term that represents all the tissues which develop from the genital ridge of the embryo. This includes ovaries, fallopian tubes, uterus, cervix, cuff of upper vagina and the round ligaments.
2. The ovaries produce progesterone, which may act as a potential antigenic hapten.
3. Gynecic tissues produce potential antigenic protein.
4. The joining of hapten and protein form an antigenic complex.
5. The antigenic complex joins with antibody to form immune complexes.
6. The immune complexes, when they react with complement, can produce irritation-inflammation anywhere in the body.
7. Experimentation has demonstrated what are believed to be immune complexes circulating in the blood at the time of dysmenorrhea that can reproduce that dysmenorrhea.
8. The surgical removal of all available gynecic tissues except one ovary reduces the ability to make potential antigenic protein to such a low level that there is essentially no postoperative gynecic immune reactivity.

MY CASE REPORTS WITH "IMPOSSIBLE RESULTS"

Ten years ago I tried to publish this information in medical journals, but my manuscripts were rejected with notations such as:

"Our neurological consultants report to us that this is impossible. I believe the author is not telling the truth!" So here are a few case reports that have already been branded as impossible lies, but I assure you that each woman is alive today to attest to her absolute personal satisfaction and to the veracity of my report. I calculate that countless thousands of other incapacitated women would have received great benefit from this information in these intervening years if there had only been medical ears to hear!

My patient Naomi Y #51 was 24 years old at the time of her final admission to the hospital in March 1981. At age 17 her left tube and ovary were removed by another doctor because of dysmenorrhea expressed as left low abdominal pain. Microscopic examination of the tissue removed revealed a corpus luteum, which is a normal ovarian finding each month. Irregular episodes of bleeding and abdominal pain besieged her with increasing intensity.

At age 19 a diagnostic D&C and laparoscopy were performed for the problem of increasingly severe pain. Positive findings were limited to bloody fluid in the pelvis that cultured negative and contained many mononuclear cells. A presacral neurectomy (nerve cut) was done at age 20 because of the severe persistent dysmenorrhea, but it failed to help. Cyclic hormones seemed to help a little at times, but for the most part seemed to aggravate her problem. Good symptom control was achieved with ethinyl estradiol (estrogen) to halt ovulation, but after a time she developed unpleasant reactions to this medication. All imaginable pain-relieving regimens were tried, using hormones, narcotics, high doses of cortisone, colchicine, etc., but without benefit. Danocrine apparently produced a temporary blindness, so it was immediately stopped.

The most severe pain, which was in her right lower abdomen, started at the time of ovulation and ceased upon the conclusion of menstruation, giving her three weeks of pain per month. A premenstrual bloat of about six pounds contributed to considerable premenstrual irritability. Nausea, vomiting and diarrhea started four days premenstrually. For many months a severe urinary bladder retention up to 1,000 cubic centimeters, with a normal bladder capacity of 500 cc, required constant Foley catheter drainage preceding and during menstruation. With several consecutive months of similar problems, hospitalization and utilization of narcotics for pain relief, she inadvertently became addicted to demerol and required a program for narcotic withdrawal.

The next stop on Naomi's unhappy trail was her introduction to a program of progesterone neutralization-desensitization administered by a medical facility in Texas. Through multiple injections of progesterone in the appropriate dosage and at the appropriate times, she was able to attain a marked improvement of her symptoms for about one year.

In April 1980, at age 23, Naomi had an episode of diarrhea and vomiting, and one week later pain developed throughout the length of her spine. The pain was worsened by activity and was accompanied by headaches. In May 1980 she developed generalized hives and also noted that her left toes were becoming numb. Examinations by internists and neurologists suspecting multiple sclerosis or Guillain-Barré syndrome gave inconclusive findings. Both numbness and weakness extended from her left foot up to her knee and thigh, and her right foot was becoming numb. An attempt was made to treat her with hypnosis, but the same weakness-paralysis persisted throughout the trance.

In June, physical therapy was administered for a left foot drop and weakness of her right leg. Splints and then leg braces were applied to the left leg. Naomi was aware that her problems of numbness and muscular weakness were of a cyclic nature with exacerbation before and during menstruation, and then some amelioration following the menses. She came to need crutches to get about. Overall, her progress was downhill, with the nerve damage being additive, especially that of the left leg, which she could no longer move or feel. The progesterone shots were discontinued in October 1980. At that time her hands were becoming numb, and she also developed sciatic nerve pain, which was explained by her uneven gait. In January and February 1981, numbness and weakness of both arms sometimes made it difficult for her to hold a glass of water or to dress herself. She developed muscular fatigue rapidly when she tried to write. She experienced muscular spasms, usually initiated by muscular tiredness. For three months she was completely unable to have a spontaneous bowel movement. The muscles of her left leg shrank markedly and pulled her left foot so sharply inward that she had to walk on the side of her foot. With the assistance of crutches, leg and foot braces and family helpers, she essentially fell from one room to another. The numbness was now rising into her face.

Naomi participated in my autologous transfusion experiment, and she was able to identify her units of blood accurately by her symptoms. This would again suggest that her problems were related to a chemical reactivity rather than to a psychosomatic process.

Examinations and consultations by internists, urologists, gastroenterologists, endocrinologists, nephrologists, surgeons, psychiatrists, neurologists and gynecologists, including professors from several medical schools, provided no reasonable answer for Naomi's devastating problem, nor were there any constructive ideas as to what should be done. It took me more than six months to convince Naomi, over the strenuous objections of her neurologist and other consultants, to accept hysterectomy as treatment for her problem. The verge of complete physical and emotional disintegration was the final convincer—there was nothing left for her to lose, and an early death by generalized paralysis was the looming probability.

My concept of the hoped-for benefit from the surgery was that the mass of her gynecic tissues would be reduced to below the reactive antigenic threshold and that this would prevent the repeated monthly episodes of immune attacks upon her gynecic tissues as well as upon the nerve tissues. I hoped that this would keep her from ever getting any worse than the best time she had been experiencing between her periods.

The operation consisted of total abdominal hysterectomy with a right salpingectomy (the left tube and ovary had previously been removed), bilateral round ligamentectomy and removal of a cuff of vagina around the cervix. Only a normal right ovary remained. There were no apparent gross or microscopic abnormalities of adhesive disease or endometriosis.

Postoperative progress: As early as the first postoperative day, Naomi demonstrated improving muscular power, decreasing numbness and improved bladder function. Normal bowel function was present after three days. By four days motor power was returning slightly to her previously totally paralyzed leg. Absent reflexes slowly started returning. In three weeks she could walk with a leg brace, crutches and assistance, but she was mostly in a wheelchair. At eight weeks she no longer needed the wheelchair and could walk with crutches, a leg brace and no assistance. After two years of physical therapy she could finally turn her left foot down so that she could walk on it without a brace. Then her shrunken leg muscles rapidly returned to normal size. Naomi thereafter walked for miles and then jogged for miles. She is now a powerful downhill skier. Four years after the operation I danced the kazatski with Naomi at her wedding. She remains in perfect health, and, though unable to bear children, she is the happy mother of an adopted child.

Naomi's medical story demonstrates dysfunctional involvement of every portion of her nervous system: central, cranial nerves, peripheral sensory, peripheral motor and autonomic. These adverse neuropathologic alterations were apparently associated with the hormones of menstruation and also possibly with the administration of exogenous progesterone by injection. I propose that the disease was caused by progesterone immune complexes. The surgery removed the very major portion of the gynecic tissues, which represent the source of the potential antigenic protein, and conserved an ovary, which represents the source of the potential progesterone hapten. Since antigen could no longer be formed, there was complete resolution of all the presenting problems. There were no therapeutic alterations or manipulations other than the physical therapy, which had been ineffective preoperatively. It therefore becomes reasonable to assume that my basic hypotheses were correct: that this was an autoimmune disease, and that the gynecic tissues were the source of the antigenic protein. I have named the condition *cyclic anesthesia and paralysis syndrome of progesterone autoimmunity* (CAPS of PAI). It would be interesting to debate whether this syndrome represents an aspect of multiple sclerosis or not.

The fact that Naomi functioned far, far better one week after surgery than she had been able to one week after menstruation during the preoperative months suggests that there was some constant source of progesterone in addition to the cyclic ovarian source. I suspect that constant source to be the adrenal production of a reactive progesterone by steroidogenesis. By the surgery of gynecic reduction I had unwittingly inhibited the formation of antigen from the unexpected, constant adrenal contribution of hapten as well as from the expected, cyclic ovarian contribution of hapten to the progesterone autoimmune disease. Had I, for example, stopped her cyclic progesterone production by surgical removal of both ovaries and no other tissues, then she probably would have attained my preoperative prediction of being no worse than the best day of her cycle. Her basic miserable disease probably would have persisted endlessly at her lower level of symptoms from the constant adrenal supply of a progesterone. It is also possible that, after the limited initial improvement by simple oophorectomy, there might be gradually increasing immune sensitivity and cumulatively increasing nerve damage.

I first encountered Lara P #52 at the Hastings Indian Hospital in Oklahoma in May 1991, on the day following her treatment in the emergency room with the standard antibiotics for the diagnosis of acute pelvic inflammatory disease (gonorrhea). This was the fifth time in six months that she was so treated for the problem of fever, severe abdominal pain with rebound tenderness, exquisite tenderness of all pelvic organs to touch and with motion of the cervix, and a negative pregnancy test. Bacterial cultures for gonorrhea were always negative.

Lara was 28 years old and had two babies. There were no menstrual problems as a teenager. She delivered her first baby at age 20, after which oral contraceptives produced periods every two weeks. Her second baby was born two years later, and cyclic hormones again produced menses every two weeks. A tubal ligation was performed when Lara was 23.

At age 24 Lara started with gradual, increasingly severe pain problems, particularly of her right wrist and hand, but also of her right arm and shoulder. The diagnosis by a university neurologist was reflex sympathetic dystrophy, meaning that for some unaccountable reason the sympathetic nerves serving her right arm and wrist had become unrelentingly irritated, causing pain, heat, swelling and redness. She was given biofeedback treatment with little or no benefit for a diminished circulation and lowered temperature of her hand. My careful questioning revealed that the exacerbations of her hand, arm and shoulder clearly occurred cyclically in coordination with her menses, a factor which Lara noticed, but which her doctors had dismissed as completely irrelevant! Her menstrually-associated wrist pains and her residual symptoms of weakness and numbness of the hand gradually increased. Her right hand became so insensitive to temperature and touch, that she had to use her left hand to determine temperature safety. The weakness of her right hand became so marked that she was forced to rely upon the left hand to do all her work.

A troublesome personality change, with irritability, depression and crying appeared during the past year. During the preceding six to nine months Lara experienced an appalling collection of symptoms:

- Burning pain in her abdomen, especially in the lower right side, which radiated into her back and down into her thighs. The pain had extended its duration to 17 days of her cycle, and its intensity was disabling.
- Angry emotional outbursts with violence put her husband in the hospital with blackened eyes and a broken leg. She was unable to sleep more than an hour or two for three to five days premenstrually because of mind irritability as well as her pains.
- She wore extra layers of clothing with her menses, because of chilliness, with her temperature recordings up to 100 degrees.
- She suffered severely painful intercourse premenstrually.
- Severe headaches occurred for two weeks premenstrually.
- Cyclic skin blemishes were at times intense.
- Premenstrual bloat was as much as five pounds.

She experienced seven to ten normal days after the conclusion of her menses, which were of normal flow. She detected a high degree of sensitivity to caffeine products, so she carefully avoided them.

My examination of Lara showed marked abdominal and pelvic tenderness. Fluid from the vagina showed *no* inflammatory cells, which made the diagnosis of pelvic inflammatory disease unlikely. Her right hand was cold and very weak. There was tenderness of her wrist. My diagnosis was cyclic anesthesia and paralysis syndrome of progesterone autoimmunity (CAPS of PAI) along with PMS.

Upon surgery in May 1991 there were no significant gross or microscopic abnormalities other than the clips which had been applied for tubal ligation. There was no evidence for infection past or present. I surgically removed the total uterus along with a cuff of vagina, the right tube and ovary, the left tube, and both round ligaments out to the inguinal ring. The left ovary was conserved.

On the *second* postoperative day Lara reported that her right hand felt normal in temperature, her ability to feel things was improved about 90 percent, the muscular power of her hand was improved at least 80 percent, and there was no pain or swelling of the hand. Her irritability and anger were completely relieved, even though this was the most symptomatic time of her usual cycle. The abdominal pain experienced preoperatively was clearly more intense than that experienced postoperatively, an observation supported by her taking less pain medication postoperatively.

At the time of the six-week checkup, Lara reported 90 percent normal right hand sensory function, 90 percent normal motor strength, and 100 percent normal hand temperature. There were no pains, swelling or redness of the hand, wrist, arm or shoulder, and there was no pain of the abdomen, back or thighs. Emotional responses were all appropriate, with no feelings of unexplained irritability or anger. There were no intervals of insomnia. There were no febrile episodes, and there was no bloat or other evidence of cyclic activity.

Though the correct diagnostic name for this wrist condition might have been reflex sympathetic dystrophy, Raynaud's disease, or cyclic anesthesia and paralysis syndrome, over four years of previous university medical center management produced only increasing disability for Lara. The repeating diagnosis of gonorrhea with appropriate therapy proved to be incorrect. Her outbursts of violence were undiagnosed and untreated except for the lawyers handling her divorce proceedings. Because of my previous experience with this type of cyclic problem, the true diagnosis of CAPS and PMS was obvious to me, and the favorable results from the correct therapy of surgical gynecic reduction verified my concept within 48 hours. By whatever name, all the challenging conditions represented progesterone autoimmune disease.

The most reliable clue to the CAPS diagnosis and etiology is that it occurs cyclically in coordination with the menses. A secondary diagnostic clue is that usually, but not always, there are also accompanying abnormal menstrual features of PMS. The PMS did not start in Lara until three years after the wrist problem, but the cyclic nature of the manifestations was there from the very beginning.

Lara again demonstrated improvement of symptoms within 48 hours after surgery that exceeded any improvement in any cycle in the many preceding months. Again, the constant supply of progesterone would have to be of adrenal origin for the persistent symptoms, and from the ovaries for the cyclic exacerbations. The speedy relief of symptoms is in keeping with the short duration of symptoms after the introduction of immune complexes in my transfusion experiment. Had Lara's ovaries alone been removed, I suspect that the CAPS would have persisted in a much modified and steady manner, since the gynecic tissues would still be present to react with the constant supply of adrenal progesterone.

At first glance, it might seem unreasonable to do a hysterectomy for an isolated CAPS of the wrist, but I believe that transforming a painful, useless right hand into a normal right hand far supersedes any objections to removing a ''normal'' uterus.

Victoria M #53 was a 47-year-old mother of two who was a member and leader of the local multiple sclerosis support group. The diagnosis of MS had been established by several internists, neurologists and the neurology department of the medical school. At the age of 24 a suspected viral infection altered the motor function of her legs. A transient numbness of her arms and one brief episode of double vision occurred at that time. A spinal tap revealed abnormalities suggestive of irritation. She had a great deal of trouble managing her legs for walking. At age 35 an ACTH therapy (cortisol stimulation) afforded some temporary relief for about nine months. A brief episode of right facial paralysis and double vision occurred at age 40. A spinal electrode was implanted at age 42 that was intended to help her MS, but this turned out to be ineffective.

Cyclic exacerbations of her bilateral leg motor disability that occurred in coordination with menstruation created an overall downhill course for Victoria. Weakness, tiredness and increased difficulty in moving her legs started one week before menstruation, peaked two days before menstruation, and lasted until the conclusion of menstruation. The one relatively good week in her cycle was that which followed menstruation. The weakness and stiffness of her legs and thighs often extended up into her hips. Upon the majority of mornings she woke up with generalized body stiffness, along with marked aching of her muscles and joints, and this was attributed to arthritis. During the night, when she wanted to roll over in bed, it was necessary to awaken her husband to push her over, because of her constant immobility. Her muscular problems were such that she required a motorized wheelchair, walking canes and manual assistance for two weeks or more of her cycle. Residual weakness and stiffness during the rest of the time made her need support for even walking across a room. Physical therapy over the course of years had been of questionable value. Cyclic menstrual pain of variable intensity affected her back, hips and legs, and at times mimicked a ruptured spinal disc and sciatica. Numbness of her feet occurred only at the time of menstruation. There was considerable premenstrual bloating and emotional irritability.

Examination showed Victoria to be just barely able to shuffle-walk a few steps with a cane and an assistant's arm. She lacked good balance. Pain and touch perception of the legs were diminished up to the knees. The leg muscles felt soft with relaxation, but they became unusually stiff with attempted motion. Pelvic examination was entirely normal.

I surgically removed an apparently normal uterus, tubes and ovaries in July 1982. The only unusual feature I could see was a small patch of endometriosis on her right lateral pelvic wall.

By the third postoperative day, Victoria noted that all arthritic pains were gone, the sciatic pain was gone and the muscles were looser than her normal. By one week she could turn herself over in bed. In two weeks she went shopping on her feet for the first time in ten years. At six weeks she could walk without braces and walked across the room without assistance for the first time in twenty years. At seventeen weeks she could walk anywhere without support, but had to walk very slowly because of persistent muscle stiffness.

In the following eight years, Victoria maintained and enjoyed the progress that was attained by the gynecic reduction. There were no arthritic discomforts at all, and there was nothing to suggest sciatica or spinal disc problems. Muscular stiffness kept her walking very slowly. However, in 1990 at the age of 55, Victoria fell and sustained a non-displaced fracture of her arm. Within just a few days there was a marked return of the leg stiffness and weakness to the point of wheelchair immobility. A ten-day course of prednisone made a dramatic 66 percent improvement, but that improvement slowly slips away with the immune/inflammatory stress of each respiratory infection. Her doctors offer no additional treatment.

Relative to Victoria's problem, I think it is important to inform the lay reader that the tone and action of the skeletal muscles is under the control of at least two sets of motor neurons (nerves). One set of neurons, called the upper motor neurons (UMN), originates in the motor cortex of the brain and goes down the spinal cord to where a second set of motor neurons, the lower motor neurons (LMN), relays the messages to the muscle. If the function of the UMN is impeded, it results in stiffness of the muscle for which it had messages. The more the UMNs are knocked out, the stiffer the muscles become. If the UMN is killed, the stiffness becomes permanent. If an UMN is out of function because it is sick and then recuperates, the stiffness goes away. A good portion of Victoria's stiffness went away because many UMNs got better, but also many UMNs apparently died, because they had been sick for more than twenty years. Multiple sclerosis has a prominent effect upon the UMNs.

If the LMN is put out of action, there is a weakness that may progress to paralysis, and the muscle will atrophy or shrink until the time the LMN recuperates. If the LMN dies, there will be no recuperation of the muscle. Remember that in Victoria the prominent loss was UMNs with stiffness, while in Naomi and Lara the predominant temporary loss was LMNs with vulnerability to paralysis along with muscle shrinkage.

Victoria demonstrated many areas of nerve damage and irritation which produced a multiplicity of symptoms. We could assign to her the diagnoses of multiple sclerosis, cyclic anesthesia and paralysis syndrome, peripheral polyneuropathy, spinal disc, sciatica and PMS with tension. The hysterectomy and removal of the tubes and ovaries somehow or other caused *all* of these problems to either disappear or improve remarkably. That strongly suggests that all the abnormalities were of the same etiology, which I believe was the adverse antigenic function of the genital ridge-derived tissues for many years. When the production of potential antigenic protein is stopped, there will be no immune reaction. There is just one common source for the protein, but there are two sources for the reactive haptens, the ovaries and the adrenals.

In retrospect, with greater experience and with further Monday-morning analysis, I believe I made an erroneous decision in Victoria's surgery . I did not remove the round ligaments and a good cuff of vagina, because at that time I mistakenly believed that removal of the ovaries would forever end the progesterone problem. I also failed to take her tiny patch of endometriosis into account, and that now represents to me a more intense immune reactivity. The incomplete gynecic reduction allowed an increased possibility of future stresses reactivating the gynecic process of producing potential antigenic protein, which could combine with adrenal progesterone.

I have another patient, Jenny N #53, who had cyclic anesthesia paralysis only during menstruation. For the remainder of each month she was perfect, with no residual symptoms as the three previously cited patients experienced. Why did her problem turn off completely? You guessed it—because there was *no adrenal* contribution of a reactive form of progesterone. How did I save her from having to pull her body across the floor each period time with her arms as her legs dragged behind? You guessed it again—hysterectomy with gynecic reduction and conservation of one ovary.

I would like to speculate about the character of the adrenal hapten, which in all likelihood is steroidal. First, its presence has not been proven, but my deductive speculation places it there. It must be similar to progesterone in order to occupy the same binding sites, but it must also be slightly different from progesterone, because it does not duplicate all of its actions. If it did duplicate exactly, there would be constant premenstrual tension, which I have never observed. The adrenal influence seems to be slightly more toxic to the target cells, and that could be due to constant irritation, a greater quantity, or a greater irritational effect of that particularly formed immune complex.

The preceding cases with cyclic anesthesia and paralysis accentuate the paralysis and minimize the arthritis. I now present another case report which strengthens the arthritis connection with the gynecic tissues. These cases are used to demonstrate clearly the powerful basic mechanism of the uterine-gynecic physiology which can be present without demonstrable microscopic uterine pathology. Most commonly the minor problems can be handled medically, but sometimes surgery becomes a must.

Maria G #55 was 45 years old wen she first came to see me for a problem of severe dysmenorrhea, moderate menorrhagia, five to six pounds of premenstrual bloat and moderate menstrual emotional irritability. Of greater distress to Maria was her rheumatoid arthritis that affected many joints and muscles with pain, stiffness and swelling. Her toes became too swollen for her shoes and she was unable to wiggle them even slightly. She hurt very much at rest, but she cried many tears whenever it was necessary for her to move, especially when negotiating stairs. She was caring for her husband and three children inadequately because of her arthritis pains. Marie's rheumatologist was unable to improve her pain status.

Maria's menstrual problems encompassed 2.5 to 3 weeks of her 4 week cycle. Of importance, the intensity of her arthritis pains also fluctuated about 30 percent in coordination with her menses. The use of cyclic estrogen and progestins produced only slight overall improvements, and she was still left with disabling pains.

My examination revealed many swollen and tender joints. Abdominal and pelvic exam revealed no unusual feature other than right lower abdominal and right pelvic tenderness. No cysts or tumors were detectable.

Maria's operation consisted of total hysterectomy with removal of a cuff of vagina, both tubes, ovaries and round ligaments. There were no significant microscopic abnormalities. Marie's recuperation was assisted by cyclic Premarin 1.25 mg. Obviously her menstrual problems were gone 100 percent. I expected her arthritis would improve 30 percent, but by surprise she was 60 percent better. Was this again adrenal influence? Five days after surgery she could wriggle her toes again as the swelling disappeared. Her rheumatologist would not visit her in protest to what I did!

Maria was pleased with the marked improvement in her life, but she was still hurting unpleasantly. Her visit to an Indian doctor, an M.D. who worked with Indian herbs, brought her pain improvement to about 95 percent with tincture of fern.

The "Unnecessary" Hysterectomy

The subject of hysterectomy is a tense one for laymen, doctors, peer review boards and money-saving HMOs. It has been generally assumed that a hysterectomy for a uterus that contains neither gross nor microscopic evidence for disease has been done unnecessarily. That viewpoint covers only the microscopic aspects of the judging pathologist and completely overlooks the devastating biochemical and physiological effects the gynecic system can have on the remainder of the body—no thought for the intense autoimmune manifestations the patient must endure. The biochemical nature of this immune symptomatology was clearly demonstrated by my autologous transfusion experiments which dissociated the symptoms from the uterine histopathology. Very, very characteristically, these multitudinous immune manifestations are cyclic and in coordination with the menstrual cycle, and may involve one, two or three weeks of the cycle, with the good week (there must be one good week to differentiate it from a constant, nongynecic problem) being the week following menstruation.

The problem is that doctors have difficulty believing what they cannot see, feel or confirm by a laboratory test or microscope. I quantified my invisible findings by never saying "You must have a hysterectomy!" but "I believe I can relieve your problem if it bothers you sufficiently to have an abdominal hysterectomy. You must make up your own mind if it is worth it to you." No rational person will undergo an abdominal hysterectomy for a minimal problem, but all too often the nonhurting medical system takes the decision away from the severely distressed patient.

A very common problem is emotional irritability whereby the women become anything from grumpy to depressed to violent, as in LP #52. Hysterectomy solved several cyclic alcoholic problems. A woman who aspired to be a bank president realized that she could never get there with her periodic sobbing at the board meetings—solved by hysterectomy. As patient NY #24 had cyclic urinary retention, other women have cyclic urinary incontinence. I have controlled cyclic epileptiform convulsions, monthly "influenza" with fevers to 103, cyclic asthma, cyclic headaches and backaches. Women experience cyclic deafness, anosmia, visual problems and inability to think. These problems have been unfairly attributed to female hysteria. These poor souls shop around from doctor to doctor, because no one will listen, understand or take requested action (hysterectomy) in their behalf. And now we have the CAPS syndrome which nobody understands!

I am quite certain that if I were to call up an HMO nurse today to beg permission to do a hysterectomy for a paralyzed hand as in LP #52, permission and payment would be refused, but if I called to remove a fibroid tumor, my request would be automatically accepted, even though the fibroid was producing no problems other than not contributing to my income.

The new system for ablating the endometrium to stop the problem of bleeding is a temporary stop-gap for many, but I believe it will balance out as an emotional devastation to women as the HMOs save money. I predict that in another five years those ablated patients will have a marked increase of their immune reactions, and at that time, since there is no accompanying bleeding, they can't possibly qualify for hysterectomy!! There is a usual combination of pain, bleeding, bloating and emotional irritability, and the only part that doctors see is the bleeding. Even women gynecologists are trained to think this way. I would hate to be a woman today in search of a gynecologist who would or could do a hysterectomy for my severe, cyclic emotional devastation. I am convinced that the only cure offered would be tranquilizers that would dope me up sufficiently so that I could no longer formulate a coordinated request, while my ability to function socially or in business deteriorated, completing my emotional destruction.

Too many women are getting caught in today's heartless, modern, medical-business financial crunch.

I conquered my hospital committees by arguing fiercely for my patients and by explaining ahead of time in the record when a normal uterus was coming out for specified physiological reasons, and I invited them to talk with my patients for verification.

Would it have truly been better for these five reported ladies to have remained cripples for the remainder of their lives to prevent "normal uteri" from being removed?

For further speculation, it is likely that the male genital ridge-derived tissues, which I call androecic (an-dree'-sik) tissues, perform very similarly to gynecic tissues in their capacity for producing auto-immune diseases. The reactive steriod would be either progesterone or testosterone, which are very similarly structured steriods (see steroid diagram page 89). The source of the steroid could be either testicular and/or adrenal. We must use the female cyclic experience to understand the more constant male performance, which could be called Male Anesthesia and Paralysis Syndrome (MAPS) instead of CAPS. The more desirable therapy for MAPS would be medical, as with GB #16. Medical therapy would include appropriate megavitamins, spironolactone and replacement progestins. When medical therapy fails, it would be reasonable for urologists to devise an androecic reduction based on embryological evidence of male genital ridge development. The big obstacle would be complete removal of the prostate, seminal vesicles and spermatic cord from their intimate association with the ureters, bladder neck and urethra. Urinary incontinence might be a common sequela to such surgery, but that might be considered a worthwhile trade for a devastating neurological disease that itself can produce urinary incontinence along with its other problems of pain or paralysis.

The most important objective of this appendix is to demonstrate to you that gynecic tissue can be the source of potential antigenic protein, which is the carrier for potential antigenic haptens which may come from the ovary or the adrenals.

I am certain that, when you purchased this book about arthritis, you never thought that you would be getting lessons in gynecology and neurology, but you must remember that arthritis is very predominantly a disease of women. Medicine is divided into many specialties, but patients are just single people that combine all those specialties into one.

Appendix B

TABLE OF FOOD CLASSIFICATIONS

FOR FOOD ELIMINATION DIET

Fruits	Vegetables	Sugar-Starch	Oils	Meat	Other
CLASS 1. Easy foods for your basic diet:					
Grape	Lettuce	Rice	Olive	Fish plain	Ample water
Peach	Avocado			Cod	Salt as
Pear	Celery			Flounder	needed
Plum	Olives			Salmon	
Prune	Parsley-flakes			Tuna	
	Cauliflower			*OR* Turkey	
	Peas				
	Spinach				
	Winter squash				
CLASS 2. O.K. foods for 48 hour add-on one by one:					
Apricot	Asparagus	Honey	Canola	Catfish	Carob
Blueberry	Cucumber	Maple Syrup	Safflower	Herring	White vinegar
Cantaloupe	Eggplant	Sugar		Trout	
Cherry	Onion	Tapioca			
Pineapple	Rutabaga				
Rhubarb	Summer squash				
Watermelon	Sweet potato				
CLASS 3. Be careful—foods for 48 hour add-on:					
Apple	Beet	Brown sugar	Sunflower	Chicken	Non-caffeine
Banana	Broccoli	Kidney Beans		Lamb	soda
Cranberry	Cabbage	Lentils		Venison	Herbal teas
Coconut	Garlic	Lima beans			
Dates	Kale	Navy beans			
Figs	Mushroom				
	Swiss chard				

CLASS 4. Be very careful—foods for 48 hour add-on:

Tangerine	Carrot	Barley	Margarine	Anchovy	Cinnamon
	Peppers	Almond	from soy	Clam	Mustard
	White	Almond	(Parkay	Scallop	Vanilla
	potato	Cashew	light)	Oyster	Spices—
		Pecan			pepper
		Walnut			M-S-
					Glutamate

CLASS 5. *Beware*—foods for 48 hour add-on:

Grapefruit	Corn	Oats	Corn oil	Beef	Milk
Lemon		Rye	margarine	Pork	Cheese
Lime		Wheat	(no	Crab	creamed
Orange		Peanuts	whey)	Lobster	cultured
Strawberry		Yeast	Peanut oil	Shrimp	Yogurt,
Tomato					Whey
					Eggs
					Chocolate
					Coffee
					Colas
					Tea
					Alcohol

READ ALL FOOD LABELS CAREFULLY

Appendix C

PREDNISONE INDUCTION GUIDE AND TREATMENT

TABLE 1

PREDNISONE INDUCTION GUIDE

Your Weight	1st week	2nd week	3rd week
100–150 pounds	15 mg	10 mg	5 mg
150–200 pounds	20 mg	12.5 mg	5 mg
200+ pounds	25 mg	15 mg	5 mg

For convenience, obtain prednisone tablets of 5 mg size only. To make 12.5 mg dosage, break some tablets in half. If the total pain score should drop to zero before the third week, immediately advance to the third week. At the end of the third week, stop your prednisone. If your total pain score has not improved ten percent or more, abandon the prednisone. If the improvement is ten percent or more, proceed to Table 2, the Pain Guide for managing the Five-day Microdose Prednisone Treatment.

TABLE 2

PAIN GUIDE
FOR MANAGING THE FIVE-DAY MICRODOSE PREDNISONE TREATMENT

Base-Line Score	(5 days off or more) Act I	(4 days off or less) Act II	Base-Line Score	(5 days off or more) Act I	(4 days off or less) Act II
0	2	3	14	19	21
1	3	4	15	20	23
2	4	5	16	21	24
3	5	6	17	22	25
4	7	8	18	23	26
5	8	9	19	24	27
6	9	10	20	25	28
7	11	12	25	31	34
8	12	13	30	37	40
9	13	14	35	43	46
10	14	15	40	49	52
11	15	17	45	55	58
12	16	18	50	61	64
13	17	19	55	67	70

Baseline Score—means your average total pain score of the last three days of your prednisone induction, or your average total pain score in your most recent week of therapy, excluding the days of medication.

ACT I—means that when your total pain score reaches this value, the Five-day Low Dose Prednisone Treatment should be started *IF* you have had five or more days off medication since finishing your last 5-day treatment.

ACT II—means that when your pain score reads this value, the 5-day regimen should be started even if you have had only four or less days off medication since finishing your last 5-day treatment. The slightly larger ACT II numbers are designed 1) to gently coax a 5-day medication rest if possible, yet 2) not let the pain score run up large numbers that are more difficult to treat.

Table 3

THE FIVE-DAY MICRODOSE PREDNISONE TREATMENT

Prednisone Dosage

Your Weight	Day 1	Day 2	Day 3	Day 4	Day 5
100–150 lbs.	10 mg	5 mg	5 mg	5 mg	5 mg
150–200 lbs.	10 mg	5 or 10 mg	5 mg	5 mg	5 mg
200+ lbs.	15 mg	10 mg	5 mg	5 mg	5 mg

For Day 2 of 150–200 lbs: *IF* the score has started going down from the first day's dosage, take 5 mg. *IF* the score has not started down, take 10 mg of prednisone.

After you have taken at least three days of medication, you may discontinue the five-day regimen *IF* the total pain score reaches baseline. The aim is to use as little medication as reasonable to attain the goal of reducing the elevated score back down to the baseline.

Appendix D

DAILY PAIN SCORE INSTRUCTIONS

THE DAILY Pain Score is designed for keeping record of your symptoms experienced and your treatments taken. One column is completed for every day of the month. Your Daily Diary should be done about the same time each day, preferably one half hour after arising.

THE DAILY PAIN SCORE will teach you to observe your body as a WHOLE rather than concentrating on your ONE worst symptom. Since you are the same person judging your same body each day, you can't really go far wrong with the number you select. *The most important thing* to be detected with time is not how much your score TOTALS, but how much your total score CHANGES from day to day in response to each therapy.

NUMBERS in the COLUMN: Enter into each of the blanks in the column below each day of the month the number which best describes the pain which you are experiencing that day in each specific joint. The following number definitions serve as a guide:

PAIN SCORE GUIDE—DEFINITION OF EACH NUMBER:

0——None (leave blank for "0")
1——Slight—no pain at rest, some on extreme bending only.
2——Slight—no pain at rest, but pain upon motion only.
3——Moderate—mild pain present at rest.
4——Moderate—moderate pain present at rest.
5——Moderately severe—troublesome pain at rest, tender to touch.
6——Moderately severe—troublesome pain, protect joint in use.
7——Severe—distressful, restricted use, loss of some sleep.
8——Severe—distressful, almost unable to use, loss of much sleep.
9——Extreme—incapacitation, immobile, no sleep.

N.B.: If a joint is painless *at rest,* (score maximum 2 when comfortable at rest), but increases to 6 with *action,* then average 6 with 2 = 4, or perhaps 4 with 2 = 3, for your score to record.

Prednisone—enter the number of tablets used that day. If a flare of pain occurs later in the day and the new pain score indicates the need for additional prednisone, enter the new total pain score and the additional prednisone in the area below the ruled lines.

Use X's to designate spironolactone and progestin use, and for the days of the FED when restricted to Group I foods. Enter each dosage strength of tetracycline. Also enter B12 shots and any helpful notes you may wish.

The Pain Score Chart is printed on the following four pages. I strongly recommend that you make several photocopies, to see you through the time of your treatment. You might also wish to photocopy the Pain Score Guide on page 241 for convenient reference.

DAILY PAIN SCORE:

Name: _____   Month: _____

Day of the month		1	2	3	4	5	6	7	8	9	10	11	12	13	14	15	16
Jaw																	
Neck																	
Chest																	
Low Back																	
Hip	L																
	R																
Knee	L																
	R																
Ankle	L																
	R																
Foot	Heel L																
	Heel R																
	Front L																
	Front R																
Shoulder	L																
	R																
Elbow	L																
	R																
Wrist	L																
	R																

Thumb	Base	L	
		R	
	Mid	L	
		R	
Pointer	Base	L	
		R	
	Mid	L	
		R	
Third	Base	L	
		R	
	Mid	L	
		R	
Ring	Base	L	
		R	
	Mid	L	
		R	
Little	Base	L	
		R	
	Mid	L	
		R	
Total Pain Score			
Prednisone			
Spironolactone			
Progestin			
Antibiotic			
FED and others			

Notes:

DAILY PAIN SCORE:

Name: _____   Month: _____

Day of the month		17	18	19	20	21	22	23	24	25	26	27	28	29	30	31
Jaw																
Neck																
Chest																
Low Back																
Hip	L															
	R															
Knee	L															
	R															
Ankle	L															
	R															
Foot	Heel L															
	R															
	Front L															
	R															
Shoulder	L															
	R															
Elbow	L															
	R															
Wrist	L															
	R															

Finger	Position	Side																	
Thumb	Base	L																	
		R																	
	Mid	L																	
		R																	
Pointer	Base	L																	
		R																	
	Mid	L																	
		R																	
Third	Base	L																	
		R																	
	Mid	L																	
		R																	
Ring	Base	L																	
		R																	
	Mid	L																	
		R																	
Little	Base	L																	
		R																	
	Mid	L																	
		R																	
Total Pain Score																				
Prednisone																				
Spironolactone																				
Progestin																				
Antibiotic																				
FED and others																				

Notes:

Selective Bibliography

These are the works I consulted most in preparing this book. Journal articles that deal with studies or with facts not generally known are cited in the test.

BOOKS

Bry A, Bair M, *Visualization: Directing the Movies of Your Mind.* Harper & Row, New York, 1978.

Chopra D, MD, *Quantum Healing.* Bantam Books, New York, 1990.

Heimlich J, *What Your Doctor Won't Tell You.* HarperCollins, New York, 1990.

Klatz R, DO, Goldman R, MD, *Stopping the Clock.* Keats Publishing Inc, New Canaan, CT. 1996.

Mandell, M, MD, *Dr. Mandell's 5-day Allergy Relief System.* Harper & Row, New York, 1988.

McCarty DJ, Koopman WJ, eds. *Arthritis and Allied Conditions* 12th Ed. Lea & Febiger, Philadelphia, 1993.

Morgan M, *Mutant Message Down Under.* HarperCollins, New York, 1994.

Rooney, TW, DO, *The Arthritis Handbook.* Ballantine Books, New York, 1993. [In my opinion, this book typifies standard medical rheumatic misinformation.]

Scammell H, *The Arthrits Breakthrough* (includes *The Road Back,* by T McP Brown, MD). M Evans and Co, New York, 1988.

Sinatra, ST, MD, *Heartbreak and Heart Disease.* Keats Publishing Inc, New Canaan, CT, 1996.

Sugrue T, *The Story of Edgar Cayce. There Is a River.* A.R.E. Press, Virginia Beach, VA 1973.

Theodosakis J, MD *The Arthritis Cure.* St. Martin's Press, New York, 1997.

Whitaker J, MD, *Dr. Whitaker's Guide to Natural Healing.* Prima Publishing, Rocklin, CA, 1996.

Wright, JV, MD, *Dr. Wright's Guide to Healing with Nutrition.* Keats Publishing Inc, New Canaan, CT, 1990.

Wyngaarden JB, Smith LH, Bennett JC, eds, *Cecil Textbook of Medicine* 19th Ed. W B Saunders Co, Philadelphia, 1992.

MEDICAL JOURNAL PUBLICATIONS AND NEWS

Annals of the New York Academy of Sciences Symposium on Aging. Vol 719, 1994.

Annals of the New York Academy of Sciences. Symposium on vitamin E. Vol 393, 1982.

Attia WM, Shams AH, Ali MKH, et al, Studies of phagocytic function in rheumatoid arthritis. I. Phagocytic and metabolic activities of neutrophils. *Annals Allergy* 48: 279, 1982.

Barnett EV, Knutson DW, Abrass CK, et al, Circulating immune complexes: their immunochemistry, detection, and importance. *Ann Int Med* 91: 430, 1979.

Beck M, Hager M, Smith VE, Living with arthritis. *Newsweek* March 20, 1989, 44–70.

Beiser SM, Erlanger BF, Agate FJ Jr, et al, Antigenicity of steroid-protein conjugates. *Science* 129: 564, 1959.

Burnet M, Concepts of auto-immune disease and their implications for therapy. *Perspect Biol Med* 10: 141, 1967.

Bush TL, Cowan LD, Barrett-Connor E, et al, Estrogen use and all-cause mortality. Preliminary results from the lipid research clinics program follow-up study. *JAMA* 249: 903, 1983.

Carter ME, Ardeman S, Winocour V, et all, Rheumatoid arthritis and pernicious anemia. *Ann Rheum* 27: 454, 1968.

Cassell G, Cole BC, Mycoplasmas as agents of human disease. *N Eng J Med* 304: 80, 1981.

Demitrack MA, Dale JK, Straus SE, et al, Evidence for impaired activation of the hypothalamic-pituitary-adrenal axis in patients with chronic fatigue syndrome. *J Clin Endocrinol Metab* 73: 1224, 1991.

Dunn AJ, Berridge CW, Physiological and behavioral responses to corticotropin-releasing factor administration: is CRF a mediator of anxiety or stress responses? *Brain Res Rev* 15: 71, 1990.

Furr PM, Taylor-Robinson D, Webster ADB, Mycoplasmas and unreaplasmas in patients with hypogammaglobulinemia and their role in arthritis: microbiological observations over twenty years. *Ann Rheum Dis* 53: 183, 1994.

Hall CA, The uptake of B12 by human lymphocytes and the relationships to the cell cycle. *J Lab Clin Med* 103: 70, 1984.

Harrigan DL, Heinle RW, Refractory macrocytic anemia with defect in vitamin B12 binding and with response to normal plasma. *J Lab Clin Med* 40: 811, 1952.

Hart R, Autoimmune progesterone dermatitis. *Arch Dermatol* 113: 426, 1977.

Irwin J, Morse E, and Riddick D, Dysmenorrhea induced by autologous transfusion. *Obstet Gynecol* 58: 286, 1981.

Jeurissen MEC, Boerbooms AMT, van de Putte LBA, et all, Influence of methotrexate and azathioprene on radiological progression in rheumatoid arthritis. *Ann Int Med* 114: 999, 1991.

King AS, Herpes zoster, *N Z Med J* 105: 135, 1992.

Kirkpatrick RA, Witchcraft and lupus erythematosis. *JAMA* May 15, 1981, pp 1937–1938.

Loriaux DL, Spironolactone and endocrine dysfunction. *Ann Int Med* 85: 630, 1976.

Mayhew NL, Shaver C, Messner RP et all, Mononuclear phagocytic system dysfunction in murine SLE: abnormal clearance kinetics precede clinical disease. *J Lab Clin Med* 117: 181, 1991.

McCarthy MF, The neglect of glucosamine as a treatment for osteoarthritis—a personal perspective. *Med Hypotheses* 42: 323, 1994.

Ortiz-Bravo E, Sieck MS, Schumacher R, Changes in the proteins coating monosodium urate crystals during active and subsiding inflammation. *Arthritis Rheum* 36: 1274, 1993.

Palmer DG, Development of the gouty tophus. An hypothesis. *Am J Clin Pathol* 91: 190, 1989.

Panush RS, Stroud RM, Webster EM, Food induced (allergic) arthritis. *Arthritis Rheum* 29: 220, 1986.

Paris J, Pituitary-adrenal suppression after protracted administration of adrenal cortical hormones. *Proc Mayo Clinic* 36: 305, 1961.

Pernager TV, Whelton PK, Klag MJ, Risk of kidney failure associated with the use of acetaminophen, aspirin, and non-steroidal antinflammatory drugs. *N Eng J Med* 331: 1675, 1994.

Platt R, Warren JW, Edelin KC, et all, Infection with mycoplasma hominis in postpartum fever. *Lancet* II: 1217, 1980.

Reichelt A, Forester KK, Fischer M, et al, Efficacy and safety of intramuscular glucosamine sulfate in osteoarthritis of the knee. *Arzneim-Forsch/Drug Res* 44: 75, 1994.

Roan S, Rethinking approaches to pain relief. *Los Angeles Times* 1 October 1996 (citing J.F. Fries, MD).

Roos JC, Boer P, Peuker KH, et all, Changes in intrarenal uric acid handling during chronic spironolactone treatment in patients with essential hypertension. *Nephron* 32: 209, 1982.

Serafini P, Lobo RA, The effects of spironolactone on adrenal steroidogenesis in hirsute women. *Fertil Steril* 44: 595, 1985.

Shargill AA, Hormone replacement in perimenopausal women with a triphasic contraceptive compound: a three-year prospective study. *Int J Fertil* 30: 15, 1985.

Shelly WB, Preucel RW, Spoont SS, Autoimmune progesterone dermatitis. Cure by oophorectomy. *JAMA* 190: 35, 1964.

Steinberg D, Parasarathy S, Carew TE, et al, Beyond cholesterol. Modifications of low density lipoprotein that increase its atherogenicity. *N E J Med* 320: 915, 1989.

Stenberg VI, Fiechtner JJ, Rice JR, et al, Endocrine control of inflammation: Rheumatoid arthritis double-blind, cross-over clinical trial. *Int J Clin Pharm Res* 12: 11, 1992.

Sternberg EM, Hill JM, Chousos GP, et all, Inflammatory mediator-induced hypothalamic-pituitary-adrenal axis activation is defective in streptococcal cell wall arthritis-susceptible Lewis rats. *Proc Natl Acad Sci USA* 86: 2374, 1989.

Sternberg EM, Young WS III, Bernardini R, et al, A central nervous system defect in biosynthesis of corticotropin-releasing hormone is associated with susceptibility to streptococcal cell wall-induced arthritis in Lewis rats. *Proc Natl Acad Sci USA* 86:4771, 1989.

Szanto E, Hagenfeldt K, Sacro-iliitis—a sequela to acute salpingitis. A follow-up study. *Scand J Rheumatol* 12: 89, 1983.

Touw JF, Kuipers RKW, The treatment of affections of the joints with progestine. *Acta Med Scand* 96: 501, 1938.

van de Laar MAFJ, van der Korst JK, Food intolerance in rheumatoid arthritis. I. A double-blind, controlled trial of the clinical effects of elimination of milk allergens and azo dyes. *Annals Rheum Dis* 51: 298, 1992 (a).

van de Laar MAFJ, Aalbers M, Bruins, FG, et all, Food intolerance in rheumatoid arthritis. II. Clinical and histological aspects. *Annals Rheum Dis* 51: 303, 1992 (b).

Vaz AL, Double-blind clinical evaluation of the relative efficacy of ibuprofen and glucosamine sulphate in the management of osteoarthritis of the knee in out-patients. *Curr Med Opin* 8: 145, 1982.

Vidal y Plana RR, Bizzari D, Rovati AL, Articular cartilagepharmacology: I. In vitro studies on glycosamine and non steroidal antiinflammatory drugs. *Pharmacol Res Comm* 10: 557, 1978.

Index

pain
   duration of as arthritis diagnosis,
      26–27, 144
   exercise affecting, 179, 181
   factors affecting, 33, 49, 52
   flare-up of, 35, 39, 55, 109, 120
   in Food Elimination Diet, 46–47
   relation to inflammation, 29,
      153–154, 171, 190, 205, 207,
      211
   see also Daily Pain Score
paralysis, 15, 84, 227, 229
   from vitamin deficiency, 59,
      64–65, 66–67
   therapy for, 164
   see also gynecic tissue; weakness
patient, role in health care
   process, 10–11, 14, 36, 85, 119, 154,
      167, 188
phagocytes
   affect on immune complexes, 19,
      22, 28, 165, 199, 201, 210
   vitamins affecting, 63, 70, 78, 146
phagocytosis, 18, 132, 137, 194
physician, education of by patient,
      10–11, 209–210
Plaquenil, 55, 100, 195
positive thinking, 156, 158–178, 213
potassium, 87, 112, 113, 114, 122
prednisone
   case studies, 33, 47, 54, 55, 62, 66,
      101, 105–106, 117–119,
      189–195
   compared to cortisol, 25, 97
   Diminished Directions Dosage, 101,
      104, 111
   evaluation of, 7, 22, 32, 35
   inflammation reduction by, 7, 140
   Microdose therapy, 7, 55, 93,
      97–101, 102, 103–104, 111,
      130, 150, 169–170, 182–183,
      191–192, 212
   therapy with, 101–110, 167,
      188–189, 196
   unscheduled doses of, 109
   withdrawal from, 106, 117–119,
      120, 190–191
   see also Microdose prednisone
      therapy
pregnancy
   mycoplasma infection in, 143

problems with, 71, 72, 117, 160
   supplements for, 75–76
   see also gynecic tissue;
      menstruation
Premarin, 88, 91, 92, 105, 195, 231
probenecid, for gout, 127–128
progesterone
   affect on arthritis, 80–81, 93
   compared to progestins, 25, 84–85
   differences in, 82, 84, 88–90, 93
   inhibition of, 180–181
   native, 24, 80–83, 84, 95,
      218–221, 231–232
   replacements for, 25
   therapy with, 4, 23–24, 80, 106,
      130, 202, 222–224
   see also hormone; spironolactone
progestin
   affect on immune response, 82
   brand name forms of, 88
   compared to progesterone, 25,
      84–85
   daily evaluation of, 35
   therapy with, 85–94, 100, 147–148,
      156, 188, 190, 196, 232
   see also hormone replacement
      therapy
prostaglandins, 68, 70, 96, 205, 219
Provera, 83, 91, 92–93, 105–106,
      149, 195
psoriatic arthritis, 78, 197, 200
   case studies, 55–56, 78, 99,
      192–195
   see also skin
psychoneuroimmunology, 161–162,
      177, 213
   see also emotions; immune system

RAST testing, 53, 195
reflexology, 184
respiratory system
   allergic reaction in, 20, 41
   disease affecting, 150
   mycoplasma infection of, 142–143,
      150
rheumatic disease
   causes, 20, 189
   compared to dysmenorrhea, 84, 86
   etiology, 3, 15, 210–211
   self-diagnosis of, 26–27